Prioritization, Delegation, & Assignment

Practice Exercises for Medical-Surgical Nursing

Linda A. LaCharity, PhD, RN
Assistant Professor
College of Nursing
University of Cincinnati
Cincinnati, Ohio

Candice K. Kumagai, RN, MSN
Clinical Instructor
Dallas County Community College District
Dallas, Texas
Rewriter/Editor
Forte Science Communications
Tokyo, Japan

Barbara Bartz, RN, MN, CCRN
Nursing Instructor
Yakima Valley Community College
Yakima, Washington

With an Introduction by

Ruth Hansten, RN, MBA, PhD, FACHE
Principal
Hansten Healthcare PLLC
Port Ludlow, Washington

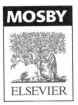
MOSBY
ELSEVIER

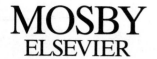

11830 Westline Industrial Drive
St. Louis, MO 63146

ISBN-13: 978-0-323-04407-3
ISBN-10: 0-323-04407-7

Printed in the United States of America

Last digit is the print number: 9 8 7 6 5 4 3 2

Preface

In these days of staffing shortages, nurses must be able to use all available patient care personnel and resources competently and efficiently. Not only must nurses become familiar with variations in state laws governing the practice of nursing, as well as differences in scopes of practice and facility-specific job descriptions, but they also must be aware of the different skill and experience levels of the health care providers they work with on a daily basis. What nursing actions can be delegated to an experienced versus a new graduate RN or LPN/LVN? What forms of patient care can the nurse delegate to the certified nursing assistant? Who should help the postoperative patient who has had a total hip replacement get out of bed and ambulate to the bathroom? Can the nurse ask the nursing assistant to check a patient's oxygen saturation using pulse oximetry? What reporting parameters should the nurse give the LPN/LVN who is monitoring a patient after cardiac catheterization or to the nursing assistant checking patients' vital signs? What patient care interventions and actions should not be delegated by the nurse? The answers to these and many other questions should be much clearer after completion of the exercises in this book.

Prioritization, delegation, and assignment are essential concepts and skills for nursing practice. Our students and graduate nurses have repeatedly told us about their difficulties with the application of these principles when taking program exit and licensure examinations. Nurse managers have told us many times over that novice nurses, and even some experienced nurses, lack the expertise to effectively and safely practice these skills in real-world settings.

Even though several excellent resources deal with these issues, there is a need for a resource that incorporates management of care concepts into real-world practice scenarios. Our goal in writing *Prioritization, Delegation, & Assignment: Practice Exercises for Medical-Surgical Nursing* is to provide a resource that challenges nursing students, as well as novice and experienced nurses, to develop the knowledge and understanding necessary to effectively apply these important nursing skills.

The exercises in this book range from simple to complex and are set in various patient care scenarios. The purpose of these chapters and case studies is to encourage the student or practicing nurse to conceptualize using the skills of prioritization, delegation, and assignment in many different settings. Our goal is to make these concepts tangible to our readers.

The questions are written in NCLEX® Examination style to help student nurses prepare for licensure examination. The chapters and case studies focus on real and hypothetical patient care situations to challenge nurses and nursing students to develop the skills necessary to apply these concepts in practice. The exercises may also be useful to nurse educators as they discuss, teach, and test their students and nurses for understanding and application of these concepts in nursing programs, examination preparations, and facility orientations. Correct answers, along with in-depth rationales, are provided at the end of the book to facilitate the learning process.

We want to thank the many people whose support and assistance made the creation of this book possible. Thanks to our families, colleagues, and friends for listening, reading, encouraging, and making sure that we had the time to research, write, and review this book. Special thanks to Ruth Hansten, whose expertise in the area of clinical delegation skills kept us on track. Many thanks to the clinical reviewers listed on the following page, whose expertise helped us keep the scenarios accurate and realistic. Finally, we wish to acknowledge our students and graduates who have taken the time to keep in touch and let us know about their need for additional assistance in developing the skills to practice the arts of delegation, prioritization, and assignment.

Linda A. LaCharity
Candice K. Kumagai
Barbara Bartz

Reviewers

Barbara Bonenberger, RN, BSN, MNEd
Ohio Valley General Hospital School of Nursing
McKees Rocks, Pennsylvania

Patsy E. Crihfield, MSN, RN, APRN, BC, CCRN, NP-C
Associate Professor of Nursing
Dyersburg State Community College
Dyersburg, Tennessee

Deborah L. Dalrymple, RN, MSN, CRNI
Professor of Nursing
Montgomery County Community College
Blue Bell, Pennsylvania

Sharon I. Decker, RN, CS, MSN, CCRN
Professor/Director of Clinical Simulations
School of Nursing
Texas Tech University Health Sciences Center
Lubbock, Texas

Tamara M. Kear, MSN, RN, CNN
Gwynedd-Mercy College
Gwynedd Valley, Pennsylvania

Patricia Sweeney, MS, RN, APRN-BC
Pennsylvania State University, Worthington Scranton Campus
Nurse Practitioner
Emergency Services PC
Scranton, Pennsylvania

Contents

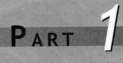

Introduction

Guidelines for Prioritization, Delegation, and Assignment Decisions

Ruth Hansten, RN, PhD, FACHE

AN OUTCOMES FOCUS

Expert nurses have discovered that the most successful method of approaching their practice is through maintaining a laser-like focus on the outcomes that the clients and their families want to achieve. To attempt to prioritize, delegate, or assign care without understanding the client's preferred results is like trying to put together a jigsaw puzzle without the top to the puzzle box that shows the puzzle picture. Not only does the puzzle player pick up random pieces that don't fit well together, wasting time and increasing frustration, but also the process of puzzle assembly is fraught with inefficiencies and wrong choices. Just so, the nurse who scurries haphazardly without a plan, unsure of what could be the most important, even life-threatening task to be done first, or even which person should do which tasks for this group of clients, is not fulfilling his or her capacity to be a channel for healing.

Let's visit a change-of-shift report in which a group of nurses receives information about two clients whose blood pressure is plummeting at the same rate. How would one determine which nurse would be best to assign to care for these clients, which client needs to be seen first, and which tasks could be delegated to assistive personnel, if none of the nurses are aware of each client's preferred outcomes? Client Apple is a young mother who has been receiving chemotherapy for breast cancer; she has been admitted this shift for dehydration from uncontrolled emesis. She is expecting to regain her normally robust good health and watch her children graduate from college. Everyone on the health care team would concur with her long-term goals. Client Orange is an elderly gentleman of 92 whose wife recently died from complications of repeated cerebral vascular events and dementia. Yesterday while in the emergency department, he was given the diagnosis of acute myocardial infarction and preexisting severe heart failure. He would like to die and join his wife, has designated a "do not resuscitate" order, and has been awaiting transfer to a hospice. These two clients are as different as apples and oranges. A savvy charge RN would make the obvious decisions: to assign the most skilled RN to the young mother and to ask assistive personnel to function in a supportive role to the primary care RN.

The elderly gentleman needs palliative care and would be best cared for by an RN and care team with excellent people skills. Even a novice nursing assistant could be delegated tasks to help keep Mr. Orange and his family comfortable and emotionally supported. The big picture on the puzzle box for these two clients ranges from long-term "robust good health" requiring immediate emergency assessment and treatment to "a supported and comfortable death" requiring timely palliative care including supportive emotional and physical care. Without envisioning these clients' pictures and knowing their preferred outcomes, the RNs cannot prioritize, delegate, or assign appropriately.

There are few times, however, in nursing practice when the choices are so apparent. All cases in acute care settings today are complex. Many clients have preexisting comorbidities that stump expert practitioners and clinical specialists planning their care. Care delivery systems must flex on a moment's notice as a nursing assistant arrives in place of a scheduled LPN; agency, float, or traveling nurses fill vacancies; and new clients, waiting to be admitted, accumulate in the emergency department. Assistive personnel arrive with varying educational preparation and dissimilar levels of motivation and skill. Critical thinking and complex clinical judgment are required from the minute the shift begins until the nurse clocks out.

In this book, the authors have filled an educational need for students and practicing nurses who wish to hone their skills in prioritizing, assigning, and delegating. The scenarios and client problems presented in this workbook are practical, challenging, and complex learning tools. The client stories will stimulate thought and discussion and help polish the higher order intellectual skills necessary to practice as a successful, safe, and effective nurse.

DEFINITION OF TERMS

The intellectual functions of prioritization, delegation, and assignment engage the nurse in projecting into the future from the present state. Thinking about what might occur if competing decisions are chosen, weighing options, and making split-second decisions, given the available data, is not an easy process. Unless resources in terms of staffing, budget, time, or supplies are unlimited, nurses must relentlessly focus on choosing which issues or concerns take precedence.

Prioritization

Prioritization is defined as **"deciding which needs or problems require immediate action and which ones could be delayed until a later time because they are not urgent"** (Silvestri, 2004, p. 65). Prioritization in a clinical setting is a process that includes envisioning clearly client outcomes, but also includes the ability to predict possible problems if another task is chosen first. One also must weigh potential future events if the task is not completed, the time it would take to accomplish it, and the relationship of the tasks and outcomes. New nurses often struggle with prioritization because they have not yet worked with typical client progressions through care pathways and have not experienced the complications that may emerge in a particular clinical condition. In short, knowing the client's **purpose** for his care, his current clinical **picture**, and the **picture** of his outcome or result is necessary to be able to **plan** priorities. The **part** played by each team member is designated as the RN assigns or delegates. The **4 Ps**, purpose, picture, plan, and part, become a hallmark for appropriately navigating these processes (Hansten, 2004).

Prioritization includes evaluating and weighing each competing task or process with the following criteria (Hansten and Jackson, 2004, pp. 163–164):

- Is it life threatening or potentially life threatening if the task is not done? Would another client be endangered if I do this now or leave this task for later?
- Is this task or process essential to client or staff safety?
- Is this task or process essential to the medical or nursing plan of care?

In each case, an understanding of the overall client goals and the context and setting is essential.

In her book on critical thinking and clinical judgment, Rosalinda Alfaro-Lefevre (2004) suggests three levels of priority setting:

- The first level is airway, breathing, cardiac/circulation, vital signs ("ABCs plus V").
- The second level is immediately subsequent to the first level and includes such issues as mental status changes, untreated medical issues, acute pain, acute elimination problems, abnormal laboratory results, and risks.
- The third level is health problems other than the first two levels, such as more long-term issues in health education, rest, coping, and so on.

Maslow's hierarchy of needs can be used to prioritize from the most crucial survival needs, to safety and security, affiliation (love, relationships), self-esteem, and self-actualization levels (Alfaro-Lefevre, 2004, p. 168).

Delegation and Assignment

The official definitions of assignment have been altered through ongoing discussion among nursing leaders. Terms such as "observation" versus "assessment," "critical thinking" versus "decision making," and "delegation" versus "assignment" continue to be contentious as nursing leaders attempt to describe complex thinking processes that occur in various levels of nursing practice. **Delegation** has been defined as **"transferring to a competent individual the authority to perform a selected nursing task in a selected situation"** (NCSBN, 1995). This definition remains as the current definition. Historically, the definition of **assignment** was "designating nursing activities to be performed by another nurse or assistive personnel that are consistent with his/her scope of practice (licensed person) or role description (unlicensed person)" (NCSBN, 2004).

Some state boards have argued that "assignment" is the process of directing a nursing assistant to perform a task such as taking a blood pressure, a task for which nursing assistants are tested in the Certified Nursing Assistant examination, and would be commonly present in a job description. Others contend that all nursing care is a part of the RN scope of practice and therefore that task would be "delegated" rather than "assigned." Other nursing leaders argue that *only* when a task is clearly within the RN's scope of practice, and *not* in the role of the assistive personnel, is the task delegated. However, this differentiation is confusing to nurses. Because both processes are identical in terms of the actions and thinking processes of the RN from a practical standpoint, the distinctions are irrelevant. Therefore, in its 2005 White Paper, the NCSBN states "using the verb *assign* in this manner (as in the above 2004 definition) is a variation of *delegation*. Since the process for both is the same, this Paper uses the verb "delegate" to describe the process of working through others and the noun "assignment" to describe what a person is directed to do (reflecting the common usage of language among nurses working in clinical settings)" (NCSBN, 2005, p. 174).

In 2005, the NCSBN altered the definition of **assignment** to **"describes the distribution of work that each staff member is to accomplish on a given shift or work period"** (NCSBN, 2005, p. 193). This "work plan" terminology is the definition of assignment used in this workbook.

Although states vary in their definitions of the functions and processes in professional nursing practice, including that of delegation, we use the NCSBN definition, including the caveat present in the sentence following the definition. Delegation is **"transferring to a competent individual the authority to perform a selected nursing task in a selected situation. The nurse retains the accountability for the delegation"** (NCSBN, 1995, p. 2). Assignments are work plans; the nurse "assigns" or distributes work and also "delegates" nursing care as she works through others.

Delegation and Supervision

The definition of delegation alone offers some important clues to nursing practice and how to compose an effective client care team. The person who makes the decision to ask another to do something (a task or assignment) must know the chosen person is competent to do that task. The RN selects the particular task, given her knowledge of the individual client's condition and that particular circumstance. Because of the nurse's preparation, knowledge, and skill, the RN chooses to render judgments of this kind and stands by her choices. Legally, the nurse is obligated to delegate based on the unique situation, clients, and personnel involved and for ongoing follow-up.

Supervision

Whenever a nurse delegates, he or she must also supervise. **Supervision** is defined by the NCSBN as **"the provision of guidance and direction, oversight, evaluation and follow up by the licensed nurse for accomplishment of a nursing task delegated to nursing assistive personnel"** (NCSBN, 2005, p. 194). The act of delegating is just the beginning of the RN's responsibility. As for the accountability of the delegates (or persons given the task duty), they are accountable to "accept the delegation and for their own actions in carrying out the act"(NCSBN, 1995, p. 3). Nursing assistants, for example, who are unprepared or untrained to complete a task should say as much when asked and could then decline performing that particular duty. In that situation, the RN would determine whether to allocate time to train the assistive personnel and review the skill as it is learned, to delegate the task to another competent person, to do it personally, or to make arrangements for later skill training.

Heretofore this text has discussed national recommendations for definitions. Although national trends would suggest that nursing is moving toward standardized licensure through mutual recognition compacts and multistate licensure, definitions still differ from state to state, as do regulations about the tasks that nursing assistants or other assistive personnel are allowed to perform in various settings. For example, at this printing, nursing assistants in hospitals do not normally administer medications, whereas in some states, specially certified medication assistants administer oral medications in the community (group homes) and in some long-term care facilities. In 12 states, statutes and/or rules have been generated that list specific tasks that can or cannot be delegated (NCSBN, 2005, pp. 178–179). Unlicensed assistive personnel are delegated tasks for which they have been trained and are presently competent to perform for stable patients in uncomplicated circumstances; these are routine, simple, repetitive, common activities not requiring nursing judgment, for example, activities of daily living, hygiene, feeding, and ambulation. In all states, nursing judgment is used to delegate less than, but never more than, the nurse's legal scope of practice. An RN always makes decisions based on the individual patient situation. An RN may decide not to delegate the task of feeding a patient if the patient is dysphagic or the nursing assistant is not familiar with feeding techniques.

The scope of practice for LPNs (licensed practical nurses) or LVNs (licensed vocational nurses) also differs from state to state. For example, in Texas and Colorado, LPNs are prohibited from delegating nursing tasks; only RNs are allowed to delegate (Hansten and Jackson, 2004, p. 77). From 23 to 28 states in 2004 and 2005 surveys did allow LPNs to delegate, but 33 allowed them to assign (NCSBN, 2005, pp. 112, 178–179). Although practicing nurses know that LPNs often review a client's condition and perform data-gathering tasks such as observation and auscultation, RNs remain accountable for the total assessment of a client, including synthesis and analysis of reported and reviewed information to lead care planning based on the nursing diagnosis. When asked whether or not LPN/LVNs are allowed to plan care or make decisions based on a comparison of the client's health data with norms, roughly half of the responding state boards said they could do so (21 of 39). A large majority of 48 state board respondents (46 to 2) did not allow LPN/LVNs to independently develop plans of care, but many (14) commented that the LPN could contribute to the care plan (NCSBN, 2005, pp. 108–109). IV therapy and administration of blood products or total parenteral nutrition (TPN) by LPN/LVNs is also widely variable by state. In all states, tasks to support the nursing process of assessment, planning, interventions, and evaluation can be allocated; however, the nursing process remains within the role of the RN. In a 2003 NCSBN-sponsored study of LPN/LVN practice (Smith and Crawford, 2004), employers at 532 hospitals, 494 long-term care facilities, and 163 home health care organizations shared their current practice policies. Fifty-eight percent of study respondents stated they regulate LPN IV practice but permit administration of medications by peripheral lines and piggybacks, 32% sanction peripheral IV push, and 28% said LPN/LVNs administered blood products (NCSBN, 2005, p. 106).

The total nursing care of the client rests squarely on the RN's shoulders, no matter who is asked to perform care activities. For more information about the statute and rules in your state and to access decision trees and other helpful aides to delegation and supervision, visit NCSBN on the web at www.ncsbn.org. Your state practice act will be linked at that site.

MAKING ASSIGNMENTS

In current hospital environments, the process of assigning or creating a work plan is dependent on who is available, present, and accounted for, and with what roles and competencies, for each shift. Assignment **"describes the distribution of work that each staff member is to accomplish on a given shift or work period"** (NCSBN, 2005, p. 193). Classical care delivery models once named *total patient care* have "morphed" into a combination of team, functional, or primary care nursing; given the projected client outcomes, the present state, and the available staff. Assignments must be created with knowledge of the following issues (Hansten and Jackson, 2004, pp. 175–177):

- How complex is the patients' required care?
- What are the dynamics of clients' status and their stability?
- How complex is the assessment and ongoing evaluation?
- What kind of infection control is necessary?
- Are there any individual safety precautions?
- Is there special technology involved in the care, and who is skilled in its use?
- How much supervision and oversight will be needed based on the staff's numbers and expertise?
- How available are the supervising RNs?
- How will the physical location of clients affect time and availability of care?
- Can continuity of care be maintained?
- Are there any personal reasons to allocate duties for a particular patient, or are there nurse or patient preferences that should be taken into account? Factors such as staff difficulties with a particular diagnosis, patient preferences for an employee's care on a previous admission, or a staff member's need for a particular learning experience would be taken into account.
- Is there an acuity rating system that will help distribute care based on a point or number system?

For more information on care delivery systems, refer to Hansten and Jackson's (2004) or Alfaro-LeFevre's (2004) texts in the references below. Whatever type of care delivery system is chosen for each particular shift, the relationship with the client and the results that the client wants to achieve must be foremost, followed by placing together the right pieces in the form of competent team members, composing the complete picture (Hansten, 2005b).

DELEGATION AND ASSIGNMENT: THE 5 RIGHTS

As you contemplate the questions in this workbook, you can use mnemonic devices to order your thinking process, such as "the 5 rights." The *right task* is assigned to the *right person* in the *right circumstances*. The RN then offers the *right direction/communication* and the *right supervision* (NCSBN, 1995, pp. 2–3; Hansten and Jackson, 2004, p. 175).

Right Circumstances

Recall the importance of the context in clinical decision making. Not only do rules and regulations adjust based on your area of practice (i.e., home health, acute care, long-term care), but client conditions and the preferred client results must also be considered. If information is not available, a best judgment must be made. Often RNs must balance the need to know as much as possible and the time available to obtain the information. The instability of clients immediately post-operatively or in the intensive care unit would mean that a student nurse would have to be immediately supervised and partnered with an experienced RN. The questions in this workbook give direction as to context and offer hints to the circumstances.

For example, in long-term care skilled nursing facilities, LPNs often function as "team leaders" with ongoing care planning and oversight by a smaller number of on-site RNs. Some emergency departments use paramedics, who may be regulated by the state emergency system statutes, in different roles in hospitals. Medical clinics often employ "medical assistants" who function under the direction and supervision of physicians. Community group homes, assisted living facilities, and other health care providers beyond acute-care hospitals seek to create safe and effective care delivery systems for the growing number of older adults. Whatever setting or circumstance you may encounter, you are accountable to know the laws and regulations that apply.

Right Task Assigned to the Right Person

The right task is a task that, in the RN's best judgment, is one that can be safely delegated for this client, given his current condition (picture) and future preferred outcomes (purpose, picture), if there is a competent individual to perform it. Although the nurse may believe it is best to personally accomplish this task, he or she must prioritize the best use of available time given a myriad of factors. "What other tasks and processes must I do because I am the only RN on this team? Which tasks can be delegated based on state regulations and my thorough knowledge of job descriptions here in this facility? How skilled are the personnel working here today? Who else could be available to help if necessary?"

In its draft model language for nursing assistive personnel, the NCSBN lists criteria for determining nursing activities that can be delegated. The following are recommended for the nurse's consideration, keeping in mind that the nursing process and nursing judgment cannot be delegated:

- Knowledge and skills of the delegate
- Verification of clinical competence by the employer
- Stability of the client's condition
- Service setting variables such as available resources (including the nurse's accessibility) and methods of communication, complexity and frequency of care, and proximity and numbers of patients to staff

Assistive personnel are not to be allocated the duties of "ongoing assessment, interpretation, or decision making that cannot be logically separated from the procedures" (NCSBN, 2005, p. 197).

Right Person

Licensure, Certification, and Role Description

One of the most commonly voiced concerns during workshops with staff nurses across the nation is "How can I trust the delegates?" Knowing the licensure, role, and preparation of each member of the team is the first step for determining competency. What tasks does a patient care technician (PCT) perform in this facility? What is the role of an LPN/LVN? Are different levels of LPN/LVN designated here (LPN I or II)? Nearly 100 different titles for assistive personnel have been developed in care settings across the country. To effectively assign or delegate, the RN must know the role descriptions of coworkers as well as her own.

Strengths and Weaknesses

The personal strengths and weaknesses among usual team members are no mystery. Their skills are discovered through practice, positive and negative experiences, and an ever-present but unreliable rumor mill. An expert RN helps create better team results by using strengths in assigning personnel to exploit their gifts. The most compassionate team will work with the hospice client and his family. The supervising nurse helps identify performance flaws and develops staff through providing judicious use of learning assignments. The novice nursing assistant could be partnered with an experienced oncology RN during his first experiences with a terminal client.

When working with students, floats, or other temporary personnel, nurses sometimes forget that the assigning RN holds the duty to determine competency. Asking personnel about their previous experiences and about their understanding of the work duties, as well as pairing them with a strong unit staff member, is as essential as providing the ongoing support and supervision needed throughout the shift. Consider the level of leadership and direction you would want your mother's nurse to experience if she was in the cardiac unit and her assigned nurse was an inexperienced float from the rehabilitation unit? Many hospitals delegate tasks only, a functional form of assignment, to temporary personnel who are unfamiliar with the clinical area.

Right Direction/Communication

Now that the right staff member is being delegated the right task for each particular situation and setting, team members must find out what they need to do and how the tasks must be done. Relaying instructions about the plan for the shift or even for a specific task is not as simple as it seems. Some RNs believe that a written assignment board is enough information to proceed since "everyone knows his job," while others spend copious amounts of time giving overly detailed directions to experienced and bored staff. The "4 Cs" of initial direction will help clarify the salient points of this process (Hansten and Jackson, 2004, p. 248; Zerwekh and Claborn, 2003, pp. 218–220). Instructions and ongoing direction must be clear, concise, correct, and complete.

Clear communication is information that is understood by the listener. An ambiguous question such as "Can you get the new client?" is not helpful when there are several new clients and returning surgical clients, and "getting" could mean transporting, admitting, or taking full responsibility for the care of the client. Asking the delegate to restate the instructions and work plan would be helpful to determine whether the communication is clear.

Concise statements are those that give enough but not too much additional information. The student nurse who merely wants to know how to turn on the chemstrip analyzer machine does not need a full treatise on the transit of potassium and glucose through the cell membrane. Too much or irrelevant information confuses and wastes precious time.

Correct communication is that which is accurate and is aligned to rules, regulations, or job descriptions. Are the room number and client name correct? Are there two clients with similar last names? Can this task be delegated to this individual? Correct communication is not cloudy or confusing (Zerwekh and Claborn, 2003; Hansten and Jackson, 2004, pp. 218–219).

Complete communication leaves no room for doubt on the part of supervisor or delegates. Staff members often state, "I would do whatever the RNs want if they would just tell me what they want me to do and how to do it." Incomplete communication wins the top prize for creating team strife and substandard work. Assumptions that staff "know" what to do and how to do it, along with what information to report and when, creates havoc, rework, and frustration, for clients and staff alike. Each staff member should have in mind a clear map or plan for the day, what to do and why, and what and when to report to the team leader. Parameters for reporting and what results should be expected are often left in the team leader's brain rather than being discussed and spelled out in sufficient detail. RNs are accountable for clear, concise, correct, and complete initial and ongoing direction.

Right Supervision

Once prioritization, assignment, and delegation have been considered, determined, and communicated, the RN remains accountable for the total care of the clients throughout the tour of duty. Recall that the definition of **supervision** includes not only initial direction but also **"the provision of guidance and direction, oversight, evaluation and follow up by the licensed nurse for accomplishment of a nursing task delegated to nursing assistive personnel"** (NCSBN, 2004). RNs may not actually perform each task of care, but must oversee the ongoing progress and results obtained, reviewing staff performance. In a typical medical-surgical unit in an acute care facility, optimal performance can be ensured as the RN begins the shift by a short "second report" meeting with assistive personnel, outlining the day's plan and the plan for each client, and giving initial direction at that time. Subsequent short team update or "checkpoint" meetings would be held before and after breaks and meals and before the end of the shift (Hansten, 2005a). During each short update, feedback is often offered and plans are altered. The last checkpoint presents all team members with an opportunity to give feedback to one another using the step-by-step feedback process (Hansten and Jackson, 2004, pp. 285–303).

1. **Ask for the team member's input first**. "I noted that the vital signs for the first four clients aren't yet on the electronic record. Do you know what's been done"? rather than "WHY haven't those vital signs been recorded yet?" At the end of the shift, the questions might be global, as in "How did we do today? What would you do differently if we had it to do over? What should I do differently tomorrow?"

2. **Give credit for all that has been accomplished**. "Oh, so you have the vital signs done but they aren't recorded? Great, I am so glad they are done so I can find out about Ms. Johnson's temperature before I call Dr. Smith." "You did a fantastic job with cleaning Mr. Orange after his incontinence episodes; his family is very appreciative of our respect for his dignity."

3. **Offer observations or concerns**. "The vital signs are routinely recorded on the EMR [electronic medical record] before clients are sent for surgery and procedures and before the doctor's round so that we can see the big picture of the clients' progress before they leave the unit and to make sure they are stable for their procedures." Or, "I think I should have assigned another RN to Ms. Apple. I had no idea that your mother recently died of breast cancer."

4. **Ask for the delegate's ideas on how to resolve the issue**. "What are your thoughts on how you could order your work to get the vital signs on the EMR before 8:30 AM?" Or, "What would you like to do with your work plan for tomorrow? Should we change Ms. Apple's team?"

5. **Agree on a course of action and plan for the future**. "That sounds great. Practice use of the hand-held computers today before you leave and that should resolve the issue. When we work together tomorrow, let me know whether that resolves the time issue for recording; if not, we will go to another plan." Or, "If you still feel that you want to stay with this assignment tomorrow after you've slept on it, we will keep it as is. If not, please let me know first thing tomorrow morning when you awaken so we can change all the assignments before the staff arrive."

As you answer the questions in this workbook, please recall the following principles.

Principles for Implementation of Prioritization, Delegation, and Assignment

- Always start with the client/family's preferred outcomes in mind. (**Purpose/Picture**)
- Refer to your own state's nursing practice statute and rules as well as your organization's job descriptions for current information about roles and responsibilities of RNs, LPN/LVNs, and unlicensed assistive personnel. (**Part** that people play)
- Student nurses, novices, floats, and other infrequent workers will also require variable levels of supervision, guidance, or support. (**Plan**)
- The RN is accountable for nursing judgment decisions and for ongoing supervision of any care that is delegated or assigned.
- The RN cannot delegate the nursing process (assessment, planning, evaluation) or clinical judgment to a non-RN. Some interventions or data-gathering activities may be delegated based on the circumstances.
- The RN must know as much as practical about the clients and their conditions, as well as the skills and competency of team members, in order to prioritize, delegate, and assign. Decisions must be specifically individualized to the client, the delegates, and the situation.
- In a clinical situation, everything is fluid and shifting. No priority, assignment, or delegation is written indelibly and cannot be altered. As the RN in charge of a unit, a team, or one client, you are accountable to choose the best course to achieve your client/family's preferred results.

Good luck with completing the workbook! We invite you to use the questions as an exercise in assembling the pieces to the puzzle that will become a picture of health-promoting practice.

REFERENCES

Alfaro-Lefevre, R. (2004). *Critical thinking and clinical judgment: A practical approach.* (3rd ed.). St. Louis: Saunders.

Hansten, R. (2004). Delegation and supervision of assistive personnel: Making teamwork work! *http://www.MyFreeCE.com*. Accessed June 1, 2005.

Hansten, R. (2005a). Relationships and results. *Healthcare Executive*. July/Aug 34–35.

Hansten, R. (2005b). Relationship and results oriented care: Evaluate the basics. Accepted for publication to the *Journal of Nursing Administration*, December 2005.

Hansten, R., and Jackson, M. (2004). *Clinical delegation skills: A handbook for professional practice.* (3rd ed.). Sudbury, MA: Jones and Bartlett.

National Council of State Boards of Nursing (NCSBN). (1995). Delegation: Concepts and decision-making process. *Issues.* December: 1–4.

National Council of State Boards of Nursing (NCSBN). (2004). *NCSBN Model Nurse Practice Act, 2004, Article III. Section 4C. http://www.ncsbn.org/regulation/nursing.* Accessed August 8, 2005.

National Council of State Boards of Nursing (NCSBN). (2005). Business Book, NCSBN Annual Meeting. Mission possible: Building a safer nursing workforce through regulatory excellence. *http://www.ncsbn.org/pdfs/V_Business_Book_Section_I.pdf.* Accessed August 12, 2005.

Silvestri, L. (2004). *Saunders comprehensive review for the NCLEX RN examination.* (3rd ed.). St. Louis: Saunders.

Zerwekh, J., and Claborn, J. (2003). *Nursing today: Transitions and trends.* (4th ed.). Chapter 10 by Hansten and Jackson. St. Louis, MO: Elsevier.

RECOMMENDED RESOURCES

Alfaro-Lefevre, R. (2004). *Critical thinking and clinical judgment: A practical approach.* (3rd ed.). St. Louis: Saunders.

Alfaro-Lefevre, R. (2006). *Applying the nursing process: A tool for critical thinking.* (6th ed.). Philadelphia: Lippincott Williams and Wilkins.

Hansten, R., and Jackson, M. (2004). *Clinical delegation skills: A handbook for professional practice.* (3rd ed.). Sudbury, MA: Jones and Bartlett.

www.Hansten.com Check for new delegation/supervision resources.

www.ncsbn.org: National Council Website with links to state boards and abundant with resources for delegation and supervision.

With special acknowledgment of and appreciation for Marilynn Jackson, RN, PhD, of Intuitive Options, Kasilof, AK, coauthor of Hansten and Jackson's *Clinical delegation skills: A handbook for professional practice.*.

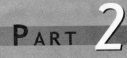
Prioritization, Delegation, and Assignment in Common Health Problems

CHAPTER 1

Pain

1. A chronic pain client reports to you, the charge nurse, that the nurses have not been responding to requests for pain medication. What is your initial action?
   1. Check the MARs and nurses' notes for the past several days.
   2. Ask the nurse educator to give an in-service about pain management.
   3. Perform a complete pain assessment and history on the client.
   4. Have a conference with the nurses responsible for the care of this client.

2. Family members are encouraging your client to "tough it out" rather than run the risk of becoming addicted to narcotics. The client is stoically abiding by the family's wishes. Priority nursing interventions for this client should target which dimension of pain?
   1. Sensory
   2. Affective
   3. Sociocultural
   4. Behavioral
   5. Cognitive

3. A client with diabetic neuropathy reports a burning, electrical-type pain in the lower extremities that is not responding to NSAIDs. You anticipate that the physician will order which adjuvant medication for this type of pain?
   1. amitriptyline (Elavil)
   2. corticosteroids
   3. methylphenidate (Ritalin)
   4. lorazepam (Ativan)

4. Which client is most likely to receive opioids for extended periods of time?
   1. A client with fibromyalgia
   2. A client with phantom limb pain
   3. A client with progressive pancreatic cancer
   4. A client with trigeminal neuralgia

5. As the charge nurse, you are reviewing the charts of clients who were assigned to a newly graduated RN. The RN has correctly charted dose and time of medication, but there is no documentation
regarding non-pharmaceutical measures. What action should you take first?
   1. Make a note in the nurse's file and continue to observe clinical performance.
   2. Refer the new nurse to the in-service education department.
   3. Quiz the nurse about knowledge of pain management.
   4. Give praise for the correct dose and time and discuss the deficits in charting.

6. In caring for a young child with pain, which assessment tool is the most useful?
   1. Simple description pain intensity scale
   2. 0–10 numeric pain scale
   3. Faces pain-rating scale
   4. McGill-Melzack pain questionnaire

7. In applying the principles of pain treatment, what is the first consideration?
   1. Treatment is based on client goals.
   2. A multidisciplinary approach is needed.
   3. The client must be believed about perceptions of own pain.
   4. Drug side effects must be prevented and managed.

8. Which route of administration is preferred if immediate analgesia and rapid titration are necessary?
   1. Intraspinal
   2. Patient-controlled analgesia (PCA)
   3. Intravenous (IV)
   4. Sublingual

9. When titrating an analgesic to manage pain, what is the priority goal?
   1. Administer smallest dose that provides relief with the fewest side effects.
   2. Titrate upward until the client is pain free.
   3. Titrate downwards to prevent toxicity.
   4. Ensure that the drug is adequate to meet the client's subjective needs.

10. In educating clients about non-pharmaceutical alternatives, which topic could you delegate to an
experienced LPN/LVN, who will function under your continued support and supervision?
   1. Therapeutic touch
   2. Use of heat and cold applications
   3. Meditation
   4. Transcutaneous electrical nerve stimulation (TENS)

11. Place the examples of drugs in the order of usage according to the World Health Organization
(WHO) analgesic ladder.
   1. morphine, hydromorphone, acetaminophen, and lorazepam
   2. NSAIDs and corticosteroids
   3. codeine, oxycodone, and diphenhydramine

   _____, _____, _____

12. Which client is at greatest risk for respiratory depression while receiving opioids for analgesia?
   1. An elderly chronic pain client with a hip fracture
   2. A client with a heroin addiction and back pain
   3. A young female client with advanced multiple myeloma
   4. A child with an arm fracture and cystic fibrosis

13. A client appears upset and tearful, but denies pain and refuses pain medication, because "my sibling is a drug addict and has ruined our lives." What is the priority intervention for this client?
    1. Encourage expression of fears and past experiences.
    2. Provide accurate information about use of pain medication.
    3. Explain that addiction is unlikely among acute care clients.
    4. Seek family assistance in resolving this problem.

14. A client is being tapered off opioids and the nurse is watchful for signs of withdrawal. What is one of the first signs of withdrawal?
    1. Fever
    2. Nausea
    3. Diaphoresis
    4. Abdominal cramps

15. In caring for clients with pain and discomfort, which task is most appropriate to delegate to the nursing assistant?
    1. Assist the client with preparation of a sitz bath.
    2. Monitor the client for signs of discomfort while ambulating.
    3. Coach the client to deep breathe during painful procedures.
    4. Evaluate relief after applying a cold application.

16. The physician has ordered a placebo for a chronic pain client. You are a newly hired nurse and you feel very uncomfortable administering the medication. What is the first action that you should take?
    1. Prepare the medication and hand it to the physician.
    2. Check the hospital policy regarding use of the placebo.
    3. Follow a personal code of ethics and refuse to give it.
    4. Contact the charge nurse for advice.

17. For a cognitively impaired client who cannot accurately report pain, what is the first action that you should take?
    1. Closely assess for nonverbal signs such as grimacing or rocking.
    2. Obtain baseline behavioral indicators from family members.
    3. Look at the MAR and chart, to note the time of the last dose and response.
    4. Give the maximum PRN dose within the minimum time frame for relief.

18. Which route of administration is preferable for administration of daily analgesics (if all body systems are functional)?
    1. IV
    2. IM or subcutaneous
    3. Oral
    4. Transdermal
    5. PCA

19. A first day post-operative client on a PCA pump reports that the pain control is inadequate. What is the first action you should take?
    1. Deliver the bolus dose per standing order.
    2. Contact the physician to increase the dose.
    3. Try non-pharmacological comfort measures.
    4. Assess the pain for location, quality, and intensity.

20. Which non-pharmacological measure is particularly useful for a client with acute pancreatitis?
    1. Diversional therapy, such as playing cards or board games
    2. Massage of back and neck with warmed lotion
    3. Side-lying position with knees to chest and pillow against abdomen
    4. Transcutaneous electrical nerve stimulation (TENS)

21. What is the best way to schedule medication for a client with constant pain?
    1. PRN at the client's request
    2. Prior to painful procedures
    3. IV bolus after pain assessment
    4. Around-the-clock

22. Which client(s) are appropriate to assign to the LPN/LVN, who will function under the supervision of the RN or team leader? (Choose all that apply.)
    1. A client who needs pre-op teaching for use of a PCA pump
    2. A client with a leg cast who needs neurologic checks and PRN hydrocodone
    3. A client post-op toe amputation with diabetic neuropathic pain
    4. A client with terminal cancer and severe pain who is refusing medication

23. For a client who is taking aspirin, which laboratory value should be reported to the physician?
    1. Potassium 3.6 mEq/L
    2. Hematocrit 41%
    3. PT 14 seconds
    4. BUN 20 mg/dL

24. Which client(s) would be appropriate to assign to a newly graduated RN, who has recently completed orientation? (Choose all that apply.)
    1. An anxious, chronic pain client who frequently uses the call button
    2. A client second day post-op who needs pain medication prior to dressing changes
    3. A client with HIV who reports headache and abdominal and pleuritic chest pain
    4. A client who is being discharged with a surgically implanted catheter

25. A family member asks you, "Why can't you give more pain medicine? He is still having a lot of pain." What is your best response?
    1. "The doctor ordered the medicine to be given every 4 hours."
    2. "If the medication is given too frequently he could suffer ill effects."
    3. "Please tell him that I will be right there to check on him."
    4. "Let's wait about 30–40 minutes. If there is no relief I'll call the doctor."

CHAPTER 2

Cancer

1. You are caring for a patient with esophageal cancer. Which task could be delegated to the nursing assistant?
   1. Assist the patient with oral hygiene.
   2. Observe the patient's response to feedings.
   3. Facilitate expression of grief or anxiety.
   4. Initiate daily weights.

2. A 56-year-old patient comes to the walk-in clinic for scant rectal bleeding and intermittent diarrhea and constipation for the past several months. There is a history of polyps and a family history for colorectal cancer. While you are trying to teach about colonoscopy, the patient becomes angry and threatens to leave. What is the priority diagnosis?
   1. Diarrhea/Constipation related to altered bowel patterns
   2. Knowledge Deficit related to disease process and diagnostic procedure
   3. Risk for Fluid Volume Deficit related to rectal bleeding and diarrhea
   4. Anxiety related to unknown outcomes and perceived threats to body integrity

3. Which patient is at greatest risk for pancreatic cancer?
   1. An elderly black male with a history of smoking and alcohol use
   2. A young, white, obese female with no known health issues
   3. A young black male with juvenile onset diabetes
   4. An elderly white female with a history of pancreatitis

4. The disease progress of cancers, such as cervical or Hodgkin's, can be classified according to a clinical staging system. Place the description of stages 0–IV in the correct order.
   1. Metastasis
   2. Limited local spread
   3. Cancer in situ
   4. Tumor limited to tissue of origin
   5. Extensive local and regional spread

   ____, ____, ____, ____, ____

5. In assigning patients with alterations related to gastrointestinal (GI) cancer, which would be the most appropriate nursing care tasks to assign to the LPN/LVN, under supervision of the team leader RN?
   1. A patient with severe anemia secondary to GI bleeding
   2. A patient who needs enemas and antibiotics to control GI bacteria
   3. A patient who needs pre-op teaching for bowel resection surgery
   4. A patient who needs central line insertion for chemotherapy

6. A community health center is preparing a presentation on the prevention and detection of cancer. Which health care professional (RN, LPN/LVN, nurse practitioner, nutritionist) should be assigned to address the following topics?
   1. Explain screening exams and diagnostic testing for common cancers _____
   2. How to plan a balanced diet and reduce fats and preservatives_____
   3. Prepare a poster on the seven warning signs of cancer _____
   4. How to practice breast or testicular self-examinations _____
   5. Strategies for reducing risk factors such as smoking and obesity_____

7. The physician tells the patient that there will be an initial course of treatment with continued maintenance treatments and ongoing observation for signs and symptoms over a prolonged period of time. You can help the patient by reinforcing that the primary goal for this type of treatment is:
   1. Cure
   2. Control
   3. Palliation
   4. Permanent remission

8. For a patient who is experiencing side effects of radiation therapy, which task would be the most appropriate to delegate to the nursing assistant?
   1. Assist the patient to identify patterns of fatigue.
   2. Recommend participation in a walking program.
   3. Report the amount and type of food consumed from the tray.
   4. Check the skin for redness and irritation after the treatment.

9. For a patient on the chemotherapeutic drug vincristine (Oncovin), which of the following side effects should be reported to the physician?
   1. Fatigue
   2. Nausea and vomiting
   3. Paresthesia
   4. Anorexia

10. For a patient who is receiving chemotherapy, which laboratory result is of particular importance?
    1. WBC
    2. PT and PTT
    3. Electrolytes
    4. BUN

11. For care of a patient who has oral cancer, which task would be appropriate to delegate to the LPN/LVN?
    1. Assist the patient to brush and floss.
    2. Explain when brushing and flossing are contraindicated.
    3. Give antacids and sucralfate suspension as ordered.
    4. Recommend saliva substitutes.

12. When assigning staff to patients who are receiving chemotherapy, what is the major consideration about chemotherapeutic drugs?
    1. During preparation, drugs may be absorbed through the skin or inhaled.
    2. Many chemotherapeutics are vesicants.
    3. Chemotherapeutics are frequently given through central venous access devices.
    4. Oral and venous routes are the most common.

13. You have just received the morning report from the night shift nurses. List the order of priority for assessing and caring for these patients.
    1. A patient who developed tumor lysis syndrome around 5:00 AM
    2. A patient with frequent reports of break-through pain over the past 24 hours
    3. A patient scheduled for exploratory laparotomy this morning
    4. A patient with anticipatory nausea and vomiting for the past 24 hours

    ____, ____, ____, ____

14. In monitoring patients who are at risk for spinal cord compression related to tumor growth, what is the most likely early manifestation?
    1. Sudden-onset back pain
    2. Motor loss
    3. Constipation
    4. Urinary hesitancy

15. Chemotherapeutic treatment of acute leukemia is done in four phases. Place these phases in the correct order.
    1. Maintenance
    2. Induction
    3. Intensification
    4. Consolidation

    ____, ____, ____, ____

16. Which set of classification values indicates the most extensive and progressed cancer?
    1. $T_1 N_0 M_0$
    2. $T_{is} N_0 M_0$
    3. $T_1 N_1 M_0$
    4. $T_4 N_3 M_1$

17. For a patient with osteogenic sarcoma, you would be particularly vigilant for elevations in which laboratory value?
    1. Sodium
    2. Calcium
    3. Potassium
    4. Hematocrit

18. Which of the following cancer patients could potentially be placed together as roommates?
    1. A patient with a neutrophil count of $1000/mm^3$
    2. A patient who underwent debulking of a tumor to relieve pressure
    3. A patient receiving high-dose chemotherapy after a bone marrow harvest
    4. A patient who is post-op laminectomy for spinal cord compression

    ____, ____

19. What do you tell patients is the most important risk factor for lung cancer when you are teaching about lung cancer prevention?
    1. Cigarette smoking
    2. Exposure to environmental/occupational carcinogens
    3. Exposure to environmental tobacco smoke (ETS)
    4. Pipe or cigar smoking

20. Following chemotherapy, a patient is being closely monitored for tumor lysis syndrome. Which laboratory value requires particular attention?
    1. Platelet count
    2. Electrolytes
    3. Hemoglobin
    4. Hematocrit

21. Persons at risk are the target population for cancer screening programs. Which asymptomatic patient(s) needs extra encouragement to participate in cancer screening? (Choose all that apply.)
    1. A 19-year-old white-American female who is sexually inactive for a Pap smear
    2. A 35-year-old white-American female for an annual mammogram
    3. A 45-year-old African-American male for an annual prostate-specific antigen
    4. A 49-year-old African-American male for an annual fecal occult blood test

22. A patient with lung cancer develops syndrome of inappropriate antidiuretic hormone secretion (SIADH). After reporting symptoms of weight gain, weakness, and nausea and vomiting to the physician, you would anticipate which initial order for the treatment of this patient?
    1. A fluid bolus as ordered
    2. Fluid restrictions as ordered
    3. Urinalysis as ordered
    4. Sodium-restricted diet as ordered

23. In caring for a patient with neutropenia, what tasks can be delegated to the nursing assistant? (Choose all that apply.)
    1. Take vital signs every 4 hours.
    2. Report temperature elevation >100.4°F.
    3. Assess for sore throat, cough, or burning with urination.
    4. Gather the supplies to prepare the room for protective isolation.
    5. Report superinfections, such as candidiasis.
    6. Practice good handwashing technique.

24. A primary nursing responsibility is the prevention of lung cancer by assisting patients in smoking/tobacco cessation. Which task would be appropriate to delegate to the LPN/LVN?
    1. Develop a "quit plan."
    2. Explain the application of a nicotine patch.
    3. Discuss strategies to avoid relapse.
    4. Suggest ways to deal with urges for tobacco.

CHAPTER 3

Fluid, Electrolyte, and Acid-Base Problems

1. A client's nursing diagnosis is Deficient Fluid Volume related to excessive fluid loss. Which action related to fluid management should be delegated to a nursing assistant?
   1. Administer IV fluids as prescribed by the physician.
   2. Provide straws and offer fluids between meals.
   3. Develop plan for added fluid intake over 24 hours.
   4. Teach family members to assist client with fluid intake.

2. The client also has the nursing diagnosis Decreased Cardiac Output related to decreased plasma volume. Which finding on assessment supports this nursing diagnosis?
   1. Flattened neck veins when client is in supine position
   2. Full and bounding pedal and post-tibial pulses
   3. Pitting edema located in feet, ankles, and calves
   4. Shallow respirations with crackles on auscultation

3. The nursing care plan for the client with dehydration includes interventions for oral health. Which interventions are within the scope of practice for the LPN/LVN being supervised by the nurse? (Choose all that apply.)
   1. Remind client to avoid commercial mouthwashes.
   2. Encourage mouth rinsing with warm saline.
   3. Assess lips, tongue, and mucous membranes.
   4. Provide mouth care every 2 hours while client is awake.
   5. Seek dietary consult to increase fluids on meal trays.

4. The physician has written the following orders for the client with Excess Fluid Volume. The client's morning assessment includes bounding peripheral pulses, weight gain of 2 pounds, pitting ankle edema, and moist crackles bilaterally. Which order takes priority at this time?
   1. Weigh client every morning.
   2. Maintain accurate intake and output.
   3. Restrict fluid to 1500 mL per day.
   4. Administer furosemide (Lasix) 40 mg IV push.

5. You have been pulled to the telemetry unit for the day. The monitor watcher informs you that the client has developed prominent U waves. Which laboratory value should you check immediately?
   1. Sodium
   2. Potassium
   3. Magnesium
   4. Calcium

6. The client's potassium level is 6.7 mEq/L. Which intervention should you delegate to the student nurse under your supervision?
   1. Administer Kayexalate 15 g orally.
   2. Administer spironolactone 25 mg orally.
   3. Assess ECG strip for tall T waves.
   4. Administer potassium 10 mEq orally.

7. A client is admitted to the unit with a diagnosis of syndrome of inappropriate antidiuretic hormone secretion (SIADH). For which electrolyte abnormality will you be sure to monitor?
   1. Hypokalemia
   2. Hyperkalemia
   3. Hyponatremia
   4. Hypernatremia

8. The charge nurse assigned the care of a client with acute renal failure and hypernatremia to you, a newly graduated RN. Which actions can you delegate to the nursing assistant? (Choose all that apply.)
   1. Provide oral care every 3–4 hours.
   2. Monitor for indications of dehydration.
   3. Administer 0.45% saline by IV line.
   4. Assess daily weights for trends.

9. The experienced LPN/LVN reports that a client's blood pressure and heart rate have decreased and that when the face is assessed, one side twitches. What action should you take at this time?
   1. Reassess the client's blood pressure and heart rate.
   2. Review the client's morning calcium level.
   3. Request a neurologic consult today.
   4. Check the client's pupillary reaction to light.

10. You are preparing to discharge a client whose calcium level was low but is now just slightly within the normal range (9–10.5 mg/dL). Which statement by the client indicates the need for additional teaching?
    1. "I will call my doctor if I experience muscle twitching or seizures."
    2. "I will make sure to take my vitamin D with my calcium each day."
    3. "I will take my calcium pill every morning before breakfast."
    4. "I will avoid dairy products, broccoli, and spinach when I eat."

11. A nursing assistant asks why the client with a chronically low phosphorus level needs so much assistance with activities of daily living. What is your best response?
    1. "The client's low phosphorus is probably due to malnutrition."
    2. "The client is just worn out from not getting enough rest."
    3. "The client's skeletal muscles are weak because of the low phosphorus."
    4. "The client will do more for herself when her phosphorus is normal."

12. You are reviewing a client's morning laboratory results. Which of these results is of most concern?
    1. Serum potassium 5.2 mEq/L
    2. Serum sodium 134 mEq/L
    3. Serum calcium 10.6 mg/dL
    4. Serum magnesium 0.8 mEq/L

13. You are the charge nurse. Which client is most appropriate to assign to the step-down unit nurse pulled to the intensive care unit for the day?
    1. A 68-year-old client on ventilator with acute respiratory failure and respiratory acidosis
    2. A 72-year-old client with COPD and normal arterial blood gases (ABGs) who is ventilator-dependent
    3. A 56-year-old new admission client with diabetic ketoacidosis (DKA) on an insulin drip
    4. A 38-year-old client on a ventilator with narcotic overdose and respiratory alkalosis

14. A client with respiratory failure is receiving mechanical ventilation and continues to produce ABG results indicating respiratory acidosis. Which action should you expect to correct this problem?
    1. Increase the ventilator rate from 6 to 10 per minute.
    2. Decrease the ventilator rate from 10 to 6 per minute.
    3. Increase the oxygen concentration from 30% to 40%.
    4. Decrease the oxygen concentration from 40% to 30%.

15. Which action should you delegate to the nursing assistant for the client with diabetic ketoacidosis? (Choose all that apply.)
    1. Check fingerstick glucose every hour.
    2. Record intake and output every hour.
    3. Check vital signs every 15 minutes.
    4. Assess for indicators of fluid imbalance.

16. You are admitting an elderly client to the medical unit. Which factor indicates that this client has a risk for acid-base imbalances?
    1. Myocardial infarction 1 year ago
    2. Occasional use of antacids
    3. Shortness of breath with extreme exertion
    4. Chronic renal insufficiency

17. A client with lung cancer has received oxycodone 10 mg orally for pain. When the student nurse assesses the client, which finding should you instruct the student to report immediately?
    1. Respiratory rate of 8 to 10 per minute
    2. Pain level decreased from 6/10 to 2/10
    3. Client requests room door be closed.
    4. Heart rate 90–100 per minute

18. The nursing assistant reports to you that a client seems very anxious and that vital signs included a respiratory rate of 38 per minute. Which acid-base imbalance should you suspect?
    1. Respiratory acidosis
    2. Respiratory alkalosis
    3. Metabolic acidosis
    4. Metabolic alkalosis

19. A client is admitted to the unit for chemotherapy. To prevent an acid-base problem, which of the following would you instruct the nursing assistant to report?
    1. Repeated episodes of nausea and vomiting
    2. Complaints of pain associated with exertion
    3. Failure to eat all food on breakfast tray
    4. Client hair loss during morning bath

20. A client has a nasogastric tube connected to intermittent wall suction. The student nurse asks why the client's respiratory rate has increased. What is your best response?
    1. "It's common for clients with uncomfortable procedures such as nasogastric tubes to have a higher rate of breathing."
    2. "The client may have a metabolic alkalosis due to the NG suctioning and the increased respiratory rate is a compensatory mechanism."
    3. "Whenever a client develops a respiratory acid-base problem, increasing the respiratory rate helps correct the problem."
    4. "The client is hyperventilating because of anxiety and we will have to stay alert for development of a respiratory acidosis."

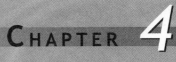
Immunologic Problems

1. You give an intradermal injection of allergen to a patient who is undergoing skin testing for allergies. A few minutes later, the patient complains about feeling anxious, short of breath, and dizzy. You notice that the patient has reddened blotches on the face and arms. All of these therapies are available on your emergency cart. Which action should you take first?
   1. Start oxygen at 4 L/min using a nasal cannula.
   2. Obtain IV access with a large-bore IV catheter.
   3. Administer epinephrine (Adrenalin) 0.3 mL subcutaneously.
   4. Give albuterol (Proventil) with a nebulizer.

2. As the nurse manager in a public health department, you are responsible for developing a plan to reduce the incidence of infection with the human immunodeficiency virus (HIV) in the community. Which nursing action is best delegated to health assistants working for the agency?
   1. Supply injection drug users with bleach solution for cleaning needles and syringes.
   2. Provide pretest and post-test counseling to those patients who are seeking HIV testing.
   3. Educate high-risk community members about the use of condoms in HIV prevention.
   4. Determine which population groups to target for education based on community assessment.

3. You are working with a student nurse who is assigned to care for an HIV-positive patient with severe esophagitis caused by *Candida albicans*. Which action by the student indicates that you need to intervene most quickly?
   1. The student puts on a mask and gown before entering the patient room.
   2. The student gives the patient a glass of water after the oral nystatin (Mycostatin) suspension.
   3. The student offers the patient a choice of chicken soup or chile con carne for lunch.
   4. The student places a "No Visitors" sign on the door of the patient's room.

4. You are evaluating an HIV-positive patient who is receiving IV pentamidine (Pentam) as a treatment for *Pneumocystis carinii* pneumonia. Which information is most important to communicate to the physician?
   1. The blood pressure decreased to 104/76 during administration.
   2. The patient is complaining of pain at the site of the infusion.
   3. The patient is not taking in an adequate amount of oral fluids.
   4. Blood glucose is 55 mg/dL after the medication administration.

5. You are completing an assessment and health history for an HIV-positive patient who is considering starting antiretroviral therapy with several medications. Which patient information concerns you the most?
   1. Patient has been HIV positive for 8 years and has never been on any drug therapy for the HIV infection.
   2. Patient tells you that he never has been very consistent about taking medications in the past.
   3. Patient continues to be sexually active with multiple partners and says that he is careful to use condoms.
   4. Patient has many questions and concerns regarding how effective and safe the medications are.

6. You have suffered a needle stick injury after giving a patient an IM injection, but you have no information about the patient's HIV status. What is the most appropriate method for obtaining this information about the patient?
   1. You should ask the patient to authorize HIV testing as soon as possible.
   2. The nurse manager for the unit is responsible for obtaining the information.
   3. The occupational health nurse should discuss HIV status with the patient.
   4. HIV testing should be done the next time blood is drawn for other tests.

7. A patient with acquired immunodeficiency syndrome (AIDS) has a negative tuberculosis (TB) skin test. Which nursing action is indicated next?
   1. Obtain a chest x-ray and sputum smear.
   2. No further action is needed after the negative skin test.
   3. Teach about the anti-tuberculosis drug isoniazid (INH).
   4. Schedule TB testing again in 6 months.

8. You are working in an AIDS hospice facility that is also staffed with LPNs and nursing assistants. Which of these nursing actions is best to delegate to an LPN you are supervising?
   1. Assess patients' nutritional needs and individualize diet plans to improve nutrition.
   2. Collect data about the patients' response to medications used for pain and anorexia.
   3. Teach the nursing assistants about how to lower the risk for spreading infections.
   4. Assist patients with personal hygiene and other activities of daily living as needed.

9. A patient who has received a kidney transplant has been admitted to the medical unit with acute rejection and is receiving IV cyclosporine (Sandimmune) and methylprednisolone (Solu-Medrol). Which staff member is best to assign to care for this patient?
   1. An RN who floated to the medical unit from the coronary care unit for the day.
   2. An RN with 3 years of experience in the operating room who is orienting to the medical unit.
   3. An RN who has worked on the medical unit for 5 years and is working a double shift today.
   4. A new graduate RN who needs experience with IV medication administration.

10. Your patient with rheumatoid arthritis (RA) is taking prednisone (Deltasone) and naproxen (Alleve) to reduce inflammation and joint pain. Which of these symptoms is the strongest indicator that a change in therapy may be necessary?
   1. The patient states that the RA symptoms are worst in the morning.
   2. The patient complains about having dry eyes.
   3. The patient has round and moveable nodules just under the skin.
   4. The patient has stools that are very dark in color.

11. A patient with chronic hepatitis C has been receiving interferon alfa-2a (Roferon-A) injections for the last month. Which information gathered during a visit in the home to conduct an interview and physical assessment is most important to communicate to the physician?
    1. The patient has chronic nausea and vomiting.
    2. The patient is giving the medication by the IM route to her lateral thigh.
    3. The patient has a temperature of 99.7°F orally.
    4. The patient complains of chronic fatigue, muscle aches, and anorexia.

12. You obtain these assessment data while completing an admission for a patient with a history of a liver transplant who is receiving cyclosporine (Sandimmune), prednisone (Deltasone), and mycophenolate (CellCept) to suppress immune function. Which one will be of most concern?
    1. The patient's gums appear very pink and swollen.
    2. The patient's blood glucose is increased to 162 mg/dL.
    3. The patient has a non-tender swelling above the clavicle.
    4. The patient has 1+ pitting edema in the feet and ankles.

13. While caring for an HIV-positive patient who is hospitalized with *Pneumocystis carinii* pneumonia, you note that all of these drug therapies are scheduled for 10:00 AM. Which nursing action is most essential to accomplish at the scheduled time?
    1. Administer the protease inhibitor indinavir (Crixivan) 800 mg PO.
    2. Infuse pentamidine (Pentam-300) 300 mg IV over 60 minutes.
    3. Have the patient "swish and swallow" nystatin (Mycostatin) 5 mL.
    4. Apply acyclovir (Zovirax) cream to oral herpes simplex lesions.

14. An HIV-positive patient who has been started on antiretroviral therapy (ART) is seen in the clinic for follow-up. Which test will be most helpful in determining the response to therapy?
    1. Lymphocyte count
    2. ELISA testing
    3. Western blot analysis
    4. Viral load testing

15. You have developed a nursing diagnosis of Imbalanced Nutrition: Less than Body Requirements for a hospitalized patient with AIDS who has anorexia and nausea. Which of these nursing actions is most appropriate to delegate to an LPN who is providing care to this patient?
    1. Administer oxandrolone (Oxandrin) 5 mg daily in morning.
    2. Provide oral care with a soft toothbrush every 8 hours.
    3. Instruct the patient about a high-calorie, high-protein diet.
    4. Assess the patient for other nutrition risk factors.

16. You assess a 24-year-old patient with RA who is considering using methotrexate (Rheumatrex) for treatment. Which information is most important to communicate with the physician?
    1. The patient has many concerns about the safety of the drug.
    2. The patient has been trying to get pregnant.
    3. The patient takes a daily multivitamin tablet.
    4. The patient says that she has taken methotrexate in the past.

17. An 18-year-old college student with an exacerbation of systemic lupus erythematosus (SLE) has been receiving prednisone (Deltasone) 20 mg daily for 4 days. Which of these medical orders should you question?
    1. Discontinue prednisone after today's dose.
    2. Administer first dose of varicella vaccine.
    3. Check patient's C-reactive protein (CRP).
    4. Give ibuprofen (Advil) 800 mg every 6 hours.

18. A patient with wheezing and coughing caused by an allergic reaction to penicillin is admitted to the emergency department (ED). Which of these medications do you anticipate administering first?
    1. methylprednisolone (Solu-Medrol) 100 mg IV
    2. cromolyn sodium (Intal) 20 mg per nebulizer
    3. albuterol (Proventil) 0.5 mL per nebulizer
    4. aminophylline 500 mg IV over 20 minutes

19. A patient with systemic lupus erythematosus (SLE) is admitted to the hospital for evaluation and management of acute joint inflammation. Which information obtained in the admission laboratory testing concerns you most?
    1. The blood urea nitrogen (BUN) level is elevated.
    2. The C-reactive protein (CRP) level is increased.
    3. The anti-nuclear antibody (ANA) test is positive.
    4. The lupus erythematosus (LE) cell prep is positive.

20. As the hospital employee health nurse, you are completing a health history for a newly hired nursing assistant. Which information given by the new employee most indicates the need for further nursing action prior to orienting the nursing assistant to patient care?
    1. The new employee takes enalapril (Vasotec) for hypertension.
    2. The new employee is allergic to bananas, avocados, and papayas.
    3. The new employee received a tetanus vaccination 3 years ago.
    4. The new employee's TB skin test has a 5-mm induration at 48 hours.

CHAPTER 5

Respiratory Problems

1. The experienced LPN/LVN, under the supervision of the team leader RN, is providing nursing care for a client with a respiratory problem. Which of the following actions are appropriate to the scope of practice for an experienced LPN/LVN? (Choose all that apply.)
   1. Auscultate breath sounds.
   2. Administer MDI (multidose inhaler) medications.
   3. Complete in-depth admission assessment.
   4. Check oxygen saturation using pulse oximetry.
   5. Initiate nursing care plan.
   6. Evaluate client's technique for using MDIs.

2. You are evaluating and assessing a client diagnosed with chronic emphysema. The client is on oxygen at a flow rate of 5 L/min by nasal cannula. Which finding concerns you immediately?
   1. The client has fine bibasilar crackles.
   2. The client's respiratory rate is 8 breaths/minute.
   3. The client sits up and leans over the nightstand.
   4. The client has a large barrel chest.

3. The nursing assistant tells you that the client on oxygen at a flow rate of 6 L/min by nasal cannula is complaining of nasal passage discomfort. What intervention should you suggest to improve the client's comfort for this problem?
   1. Suggest that the client's oxygen be humidified.
   2. Suggest that the client be placed on a simple face mask.
   3. Suggest that the client be provided an extra pillow.
   4. Suggest that the client sit up in a chair at the bedside.

4. You are supervising a student nurse who is performing tracheostomy care for a client. For which action should you intervene?
   1. The student nurse suctions the tracheostomy tube prior to performing tracheostomy care.
   2. The student nurse removes old dressings and cleans off excess secretions.
   3. The student nurse removes the inner cannula and cleans using universal precautions.
   4. The student nurse replaces the inner cannula and cleans the stoma site.
   5. The student nurse changes the soiled tracheostomy ties and secures the tube in place.

5. You are supervising an RN who was pulled from the medical-surgical floor to the emergency department (ED). The nurse is providing care for a client admitted with anterior epistaxis (nosebleed). Which of these directions will you clearly provide to the RN? (Choose all that apply.)
   1. Position the client supine and turned on his side.
   2. Apply direct lateral pressure to the nose for 5 minutes.
   3. Maintain universal body substance precautions.
   4. Apply ice or cool compresses to the nose.
   5. Instruct the client not to blow the nose for several hours.

6. The client with sleep apnea has a nursing diagnosis of Sleep Deprivation related to disrupted sleep cycle. Which action should you delegate to the nursing assistant?
   1. Discuss weight loss strategies such as diet and exercise with the client.
   2. Teach client how to apply the BiPAP machine before sleeping.
   3. Remind client to sleep on his side instead of his back.
   4. Administer modafinil (Provigil) to promote daytime wakefulness.

7. You are acting as preceptor for a new graduate RN during her second week of orientation. For which client(s) would you assign the nursing care to the new RN under your supervision? (Choose all that apply.)
   1. A 38-year-old client with moderate persistent asthma awaiting discharge
   2. A 63-year-old client with tracheostomy needing trach care every shift
   3. A 56-year-old client with lung cancer just returned from left lower lobectomy
   4. A 49-year-old new admission client with new diagnosis of esophageal cancer

8. You are providing care for a client with recently diagnosed asthma. What key points will you be sure to include in your teaching plan for this client? (Choose all that apply.)
   1. Avoid potential environmental asthma triggers such as smoke.
   2. Use inhaler 30 minutes before exercising to prevent bronchospasm.
   3. Wash all bedding in cold water to reduce and destroy dust mites.
   4. Be sure to get at least 8 hours of rest and sleep every night.
   5. Avoid foods prepared with monosodium glutamate (MSG).

9. You are the team leader RN working with a student nurse. The student nurse is to teach the client how to use a multidose inhaler without a spacer. Put the steps that the student nurse should teach the client in correct order.
   1. Remove the inhaler cap and shake the inhaler.
   2. Open your mouth and place the mouthpiece 1–2 inches away.
   3. Tilt your head back and breathe out fully.
   4. Hold your breath for at least 10 seconds.
   5. Press down firmly on the canister and breathe deeply through your mouth.
   6. Wait at least 1 minute between puffs.

   ____, ____, ____, ____, ____, ____

10. The client has chronic obstructive pulmonary disease (COPD). Which intervention for airway management should you delegate to the nursing assistant?
    1. Assist client to sit up on side of bed.
    2. Instruct client to cough effectively.
    3. Teach client to use incentive spirometry.
    4. Auscultate breath sounds every 4 hours.

11. The client with COPD has a nursing diagnosis of Ineffective Breathing Pattern. Which action is appropriate to delegate to the experienced LPN/LVN under your supervision?
    1. Observe how well the client performs pursed-lip breathing.
    2. Plan a nursing care regimen that gradually increases activity tolerance.
    3. Assist the client with basic activities of daily living (ADLs).
    4. Consult with physical therapy about reconditioning exercises.

12. The client with COPD tells the nursing assistant that she did not get her annual flu shot this year and has not had a pneumonia vaccination. You will be sure to instruct the nursing assistant to report which of the following?
    1. Blood pressure 152/84
    2. Respiratory rate 27/minute
    3. Heart rate 92/minute
    4. Oral temperature 101.2°F

13. You are responsible for the care of a postoperative client with a thoracotomy. The client has the nursing diagnosis Activity Intolerance. Which action should you delegate to the nursing assistant?
    1. Instruct the client to alternate rest and activity periods.
    2. Encourage, monitor, and record nutritional intake.
    3. Monitor cardiorespiratory response to activity.
    4. Plan activities for periods when client has most energy.

14. You are supervising a nursing student who is providing care for a thoracotomy client with a chest tube. What finding will you clearly instruct the nursing student to notify you about immediately?
    1. Chest tube drainage of 10–15 mL per hour
    2. Continuous bubbling in the water seal chamber
    3. Complaints of pain at the chest tube site
    4. Chest tube dressing dated yesterday

15. After change of shift, you are assigned to care for the following clients. Which client should you assess first?
    1. A 68-year-old client on ventilator who needs a sterile sputum specimen sent to the laboratory
    2. A 57-year-old client with COPD and pulse oximetry reading from previous shift of 90% saturation
    3. A 72-year-old client with pneumonia who needs to be started on intravenous antibiotics
    4. A 51-year-old client with asthma complaining of shortness of breath (SOB) after using a bronchodilator inhaler

16. You are initiating a nursing care plan for a client with pneumonia. Which intervention for cough enhancement should you delegate to the inexperienced nursing assistant?
    1. Teach the client about the importance of adequate fluid intake and hydration.
    2. Assist client to sitting position with neck flexed, shoulders relaxed and knees flexed.
    3. Remind the client to use incentive spirometry every 1–2 hours while awake.
    4. Encourage client to take a deep breath, hold it for 2 seconds, then cough 2–3 times in succession.

17. As the charge nurse, you are making assignments for the next shift. Which client should be assigned to the fairly new nurse (2 months) pulled from the surgical unit to the medical unit?
    1. A 58-year-old client on airborne precautions for tuberculosis (TB)
    2. A 65-year-old client just returned from bronchoscopy and biopsy
    3. A 72-year-old client who needs teaching about use of incentive spirometry
    4. A 69-year-old client with COPD who is ventilator dependent

18. You are preparing a client with TB for discharge. Which statement by the client indicates that additional teaching is required?
    1. "All of my family members need to go and see the doctor for tuberculosis testing."
    2. "I will continue to take my isoniazid (INH) until I am feeling completely well."
    3. "I will cover my mouth and nose when I sneeze or cough and put my used tissues in a plastic bag."
    4. "I will change my diet to include more foods rich in iron, protein, and vitamin C."

19. You are admitting a client with a diagnosis of rule out pulmonary embolus (PE). Client history and assessment reveals all of these findings. Which finding supports the diagnosis of PE?
    1. Client was recently in a motor vehicle accident.
    2. Client participated in aerobic exercise program for 6 months.
    3. Client gave birth to youngest child 1 year ago.
    4. Client was on bedrest 6 hours after diagnostic procedure.

20. Which intervention for the client with PE could be delegated to the LPN/LVN on your client care team?
    1. Evaluate client's complaints of chest pain.
    2. Monitor lab values for changes in oxygenation.
    3. Assess for symptoms of respiratory failure.
    4. Auscultate lung sounds for crackles.

21. The client with a PE is receiving anticoagulation with IV heparin. What instructions will you give the nursing assistant who will assist the client with ADLs? (Choose all that apply.)
    1. Use a lift sheet when moving and positioning the client in bed.
    2. Use an electric razor when shaving the client each day.
    3. Use a soft-bristled toothbrush or tooth sponge for oral care.
    4. Use a rectal thermometer to attain a more accurate body temperature.
    5. Be sure the client's footwear has firm soles when ambulating.

22. The client with acute respiratory distress syndrome (ARDS) is receiving oxygen by non-rebreather mask, but arterial blood gases still show poor oxygenation. As the nurse responsible for this client's care, you anticipate which physician's orders?
    1. Endotracheal intubation and mechanical ventilation
    2. Immediate application of CPAP to client's nose and mouth
    3. Intravenous furosemide (Lasix) 100 mg IV push stat
    4. Call a CODE for respiratory arrest.

23. You are precepting an RN who is orienting to the intensive care unit (ICU). The RN is providing care for a client with ARDS who has just been intubated in preparation for mechanical ventilation. You observe the nurse perform all of these actions. For which action must you intervene immediately?
    1. The RN assesses client for bilateral breath sounds and symmetrical chest movement.
    2. The RN auscultates over the stomach to rule out esophageal intubation.
    3. The RN marks the tube 1 cm from where it touches the incisor tooth or nares.
    4. The RN orders a chest x-ray to verify that tube placement is correct.

24. You are assigned to provide nursing care for a client receiving mechanical ventilation. Which action should you delegate to the experienced nursing assistant?
    1. Assess the client's respiratory status every 4 hours.
    2. Take vital signs and pulse oximetry reading every 4 hours.
    3. Check ventilator setting to make sure they are as prescribed.
    4. Observe client's need for suctioning every 2 hours.

25. The nursing assistant is taking vital signs for the client who is intubated after being suctioned by the respiratory therapist. Which vital sign should she immediately report to you—the RN?
    1. Heart rate 98 per minute
    2. Respiratory rate 24 per minute
    3. Blood pressure 168/90
    4. Tympanic temperature 101.4°F

26. You are making a home visit to a 50-year-old client who was discharged from the hospital 2 days ago after being hospitalized for 4 days with a right leg deep vein thrombosis (DVT) and a pulmonary embolism. The client's only medication is enoxaparin (Lovenox) 80 mg subcutaneously every 12 hours. Which assessment information will you need to communicate to the physician?
    1. The client says she has not been to the lab to have an aPTT done.
    2. The right calf is warm to touch and is larger than the left calf.
    3. The client is unable to remember her husband's name.
    4. There are multiple ecchymotic areas on the client's arms.

27. The high pressure alarm on the ventilator rings and, when you go into the room to assess your client with acute respiratory distress syndrome (ARDS), her oxygen saturation monitor reads 87% and she is struggling to sit up. Which action should you take next?
    1. Reassure the client that the ventilator will do the work of breathing for her.
    2. Manually ventilate the client while you assess possible reasons for the high pressure alarm.
    3. Increase the FIO_2 on the ventilator to 100% in preparation for endotracheal suctioning.
    4. Insert an oral airway to prevent the client from biting on the endotracheal tube.

28. When assessing a 22-year-old client who was admitted 3 days ago with multiple rib fractures and pulmonary contusions after a motor vehicle accident, you find that the client has shallow respirations at a rate of 38. He says he feels "dizzy and scared." His oxygen saturation is 90% with the oxygen at 6 L/minute per nasal cannula. Which action is most appropriate?
    1. Increase the flow rate on the oxygen to 10 L/minute and reassess the client after about 10 minutes.
    2. Assist the client to use the incentive spirometer and splint his chest using a pillow while he coughs.
    3. Administer the ordered morphine sulfate to the client to decrease his anxiety and reduce the hyperventilation.
    4. Place the client on a non-rebreather mask at 95%–100% FIO_2 and call the physician to discuss the client's status.

29. You have just finished assisting the physician with a thoracentesis for a client with recurrent left pleural effusion caused by lung cancer. The physician was able to remove 1800 mL of fluid during the thoracentisis. Which assessment information will be of most concern?
    1. The client cries and states that she cannot go on with treatment much longer.
    2. The client says that she has sharp, stabbing chest pain every time she takes a deep breath.
    3. The client's blood pressure is 100/48 and her pulse rate is 102 beats/minute.
    4. The client's dressing at the thoracentesis site has 1 cm of bloody drainage.

30. A 24-year-old client with cystic fibrosis is admitted with increased shortness of breath and possible pneumonia. Which nursing activity is most important to include in the client's care?
    1. Perform postural drainage and chest physiotherapy every 4 hours.
    2. Discuss client's feelings about the need for a living will.
    3. Place in private room to decrease the risk of further infection.
    4. Plan activities to allow at least 8 hours of uninterrupted sleep.

CHAPTER 6

Cardiovascular Problems

1. You are working in the emergency department (ED) when a patient arrives, complaining of substernal and left arm discomfort that has been going on for about 3 hours. All of these baseline laboratory tests are drawn. Which one will be most useful in determining whether you should anticipate implementing the acute coronary syndrome (ACS) standard orders?
   1. Creatine kinase-MB
   2. Troponin I
   3. Myoglobin
   4. C-reactive protein

2. You are monitoring a 53-year-old patient who is having a stress test using a treadmill. Which of these patient symptoms will require the most immediate action?
   1. Blood pressure 152/88
   2. Sinus tachycardia, rate 134
   3. Oxygen saturation 91%
   4. Chest pain level 3 (0–10 scale)

3. You are teamed with an LPN/LVN in caring for a group of patients on the cardiac unit. Which action by the LPN/LVN indicates you need to intervene immediately?
   1. The LPN/LVN assists a patient to the bathroom 30 minutes after the patient has returned from a coronary arteriogram.
   2. The LPN/LVN checks a patient's blood pressure before administering nitroglycerin (Nitro-Stat) 0.4 mg SL.
   3. The LPN/LVN returns a patient to bed after the patient's heart rate increases from 72 to 96 while ambulating in the hall.
   4. The LPN/LVN brings breakfast to a patient who is scheduled for an echocardiogram later in the morning.

4. An otherwise healthy 28-year-old woman has just been diagnosed with stage 1 hypertension. The patient is 5′6″ tall and weighs 115 pounds. She says she has a glass of wine once or twice a week and eats "fast food" frequently because of her busy schedule. Which topic will you plan on including in the patient teaching plan?
   1. Benefits and adverse effects of beta-blockers
   2. Adverse effects of alcohol on blood pressure
   3. Methods for decreasing dietary caloric intake
   4. Low-sodium food choices when eating out

5. You make a home visit to evaluate a hypertensive patient who has been taking enalapril (Vasotec) for 3 weeks. Which information indicates that you need to contact the physician about a change in the drug therapy?
   1. Patient complains of frequent urination.
   2. Patient's blood pressure is 138/86.
   3. Patient coughs often during the visit.
   4. Patient complains of occasional dizziness.

6. While completing a nursing admission history, you obtain this information about the patient's cardiovascular risk factors: patient's mother and two siblings have had myocardial infarctions. Patient smokes and has a 20 pack/year history of cigarette use. Her work as a mail carrier involves a lot of walking. She takes metoprolol (Lopressor) for hypertension and her blood pressure has been in the range of 130/60 to 140/85. Which interventions will be most important to include in the discharge plan for this patient? (Choose all that apply.)
   1. Refer to community programs that assist in smoking cessation.
   2. Teach about the impact of family history on cardiovascular risk.
   3. Educate about the need for a change in antihypertensive therapy.
   4. Assist in reducing the stress associated with her cardiovascular risk.

7. You are the charge nurse for the coronary care step-down unit. Which patient is best to assign to an RN who has floated for the day from the general medical-surgical unit?
   1. Patient requiring discharge teaching about coronary artery stenting prior to going home with spouse today
   2. Patient receiving IV furosemide (Lasix) to treat acute left ventricular failure.
   3. Patient just transferred from the radiology department after a coronary angioplasty
   4. Patient just admitted with unstable angina and who has orders for a heparin infusion and aspirin

8. At 9:00 PM, you admit a 63-year-old with a diagnosis of acute myocardial infraction (AMI) to the ED. The physician is considering the use of fibrinolytic therapy with tissue plasminogen activator (tPA, alteplase [Activase]). Which information is most important to communicate to the physician?
   1. The patient was treated with alteplase about 8 months ago.
   2. The patient takes famotidine (Pepcid) for esophageal reflux.
   3. The patient has T wave inversions on the 12-lead ECG.
   4. The patient has had continuous chest pain since 1:00 PM.

9. You are working with an experienced nursing assistant and LPN/LVN in caring for a group of patients. You have developed a nursing diagnosis of Activity Intolerance related to fatigue and chest pain for a patient who had an acute myocardial infarction 3 days ago. Which of these nursing activities included in the care plan is best delegated to the LPN/LVN?
   1. Administer nitroglycerin (Nitro-Stat) if chest discomfort occurs during patient activities.
   2. Monitor pulse, blood pressure, and oxygen saturation before and after patient ambulation.
   3. Teach the patient energy conservation techniques to decrease myocardial oxygen demand.
   4. Explain the rationale for alternating rest periods with exercise to the patient and family.

10. You are working in the ED caring for a patient who was just admitted with left anterior chest pain, possible unstable angina or myocardial infarction. Which nursing activity will you accomplish first?
    1. Auscultate heart sounds.
    2. Administer sublingual nitroglycerin.
    3. Insert an IV catheter.
    4. Obtain a brief patient health history.

11. An elderly patient on the coronary step-down unit tells you that he does not want to take the ordered docusate sodium (Colace) because he does not have any problems with constipation. Which intervention is most appropriate?
    1. Document the medication on the patient's chart as "refused."
    2. Mix the medication with food and administer it.
    3. Explain that his decreased activity level may cause constipation.
    4. Reinforce that the physician has ordered the Colace for a reason.

12. You have given morphine sulfate 4 mg IV to a patient who is having an AMI. When evaluating the response 5 minutes after giving the medication, which of these data indicate a need for immediate further action?
    1. The blood pressure decreases from 114/65 to 106/58.
    2. The respiratory rate drops from 18 to 12 breaths/minute.
    3. The patient complains of feeling lightheaded and dizzy.
    4. The patient still has chest pain at a level 1 (0–10 scale).

13. You are preparing to implement discharge teaching about heart healthy diet and activity levels for a patient who has had a myocardial infarction and her husband. The patient says, "I don't see why I need to listen to this information. I don't think that I will need to make any changes right now in my lifestyle." Which response is most appropriate?
    1. "Do you think your family may want you to make some lifestyle changes?"
    2. "Can you tell me why you don't feel like you need to make any changes?"
    3. "You are still in the stage of denial, but you will want this information later on."
    4. "Even if you don't want to change, it's important that you have this teaching."

14. You are caring for a hospitalized patient with heart failure who is receiving captopril (Capoten) and spironolactone (Aldactone). Which laboratory value will be most important to monitor?
    1. Sodium
    2. Blood urea nitrogen (BUN)
    3. Potassium
    4. Alkaline phosphatase (ALP)

15. A patient with atrial fibrillation is ambulating in the hallway on the coronary step-down unit and suddenly tells you, "I feel really dizzy." Which action should you take first?
    1. Help the patient to sit down.
    2. Check the patient's apical pulse.
    3. Take the patient's blood pressure.
    4. Have the patient breathe deeply.

16. At 10:00 AM, a patient receives a new order for transesophageal echocardiography (TEE) as soon as possible. Which action will you take first?
    1. Make the patient NPO.
    2. Teach the patient about the procedure.
    3. Start an intravenous line.
    4. Attach the patient to a cardiac monitor.

17. You assess a patient who has just returned to the recovery area after having a coronary arteriogram. Which of these data is of most concern?
    1. Blood pressure is 144/78.
    2. Pedal pulses are palpable at +1.
    3. Left groin has a 3-cm ecchymotic area.
    4. Apical pulse is 122 and regular.

18. You are working in an outpatient clinic where many vascular diagnostic tests are performed. Which of these tasks associated with vascular testing will be most appropriate to delegate to an experienced nursing assistant?
    1. Measure ankle and brachial pressures for a patient having the ankle-brachial index calculated.
    2. Check blood pressure and pulse every 10 minutes for a patient who is having exercise testing.
    3. Take an allergy history for a patient who is scheduled for left leg contrast venography.
    4. Provide brief patient teaching for a patient who will have a right subclavian vein Doppler study.

19. While working on the cardiac step-down unit, you are precepting a new graduate RN who has been in a 6-week orientation program. Which of these patients will be best to assign to the new graduate?
    1. A 19-year-old with rheumatic fever who needs discharge teaching prior to going home with a roommate today
    2. A 33-year-old admitted a week ago with endocarditis who will be receiving ceftizoxime (Cefizox) 2 g IV
    3. A 50-year-old with newly diagnosed stable angina who has many questions about medications and nursing care
    4. A 75-year-old who has just been transferred to the unit after having coronary artery bypass grafting yesterday

20. You are observing the cardiac rhythms for patients in the coronary care unit. Which of these patients will need immediate intervention?
    1. A patient admitted with heart failure who has atrial fibrillation with a rate of 88 while at rest
    2. A patient with a newly implanted demand ventricular pacemaker, who has occasional periods of sinus rhythm, rate 90 to 100
    3. A patient who has just arrived on the unit with an acute MI and has sinus rhythm, rate 76, with frequent premature ventricular contractions
    4. A patient who recently started taking atenolol (Tenormin) and has a first-degree heart block, rate 58

21. A diagnosis of ventricular fibrillation is identified for an unresponsive 50-year-old patient who has just arrived in the ED. Which action will you take first?
    1. Defibrillate at 200 Joules.
    2. Start cardiopulmonary resuscitation (CPR).
    3. Administer epinephrine (Adrenalin) 1 mg IV.
    4. Intubate and manually ventilate.

22. Two weeks ago, a 63-year-old patient with heart failure received a new prescription for carvedilol (Coreg) 3.125 mg orally. Upon evaluation in the outpatient clinic you find these symptoms. Which is of most concern?
    1. Complaints of increased fatigue and dyspnea
    2. Weight increase of 0.5 kg in 2 weeks
    3. Bibasilar crackles audible in the posterior chest
    4. Sinus bradycardia, rate 50, as evidenced by ECG

23. You have just received change-of-shift report about these patients on the coronary step down unit. Which one will you assess first?
    1. A 26-year-old with heart failure caused by congenital mitral stenosis who is scheduled for balloon valvuloplasty later today
    2. A 45-year-old with constrictive cardiomyopathy who developed acute dyspnea and agitation about 1 hour before the shift change
    3. A 56-year-old who had a coronary angioplasty and stent placement yesterday and has complained of occasional chest pain since the procedure
    4. A 77-year-old who transferred from intensive care 2 days ago after coronary artery bypass grafting and has a temperature of 100.6°F

24. As the charge nurse in a long-term-care (LTC) facility that has RN, LPN/LVN, and nursing assistant staff members, you have developed a plan for ongoing assessment of all residents with a diagnosis of heart failure. Which of these activities included in the plan is most appropriate to delegate to an LPN/LVN team leader?
    1. Weigh all residents with heart failure each morning.
    2. Listen to lung sounds and check for edema weekly.
    3. Review all heart failure medications with residents every month.
    4. Update activity plans for residents with heart failure every quarter.

25. During a home visit to an 88-year-old patient who is taking digoxin (Lanoxin) 0.25 mg daily to help control the rate of atrial fibrillation, you obtain this assessment information. Which assessment indicates that you need to notify the physician?
    1. The patient's apical pulse is 68 and very irregular.
    2. The patient takes the digoxin with meals.
    3. The patient's vision is becoming "fuzzy."
    4. The patient has lung crackles that clear after coughing.

26. You are ambulating a cardiac surgery patient who has telemetry cardiac monitoring when another staff member tells you that the patient has developed a supraventricular tachycardia with a rate of 146 beats per minute. In which order will you take these actions?
    1. Call the patient's physician.
    2. Have the patient sit down.
    3. Check the patient's blood pressure.
    4. Administer oxygen by nasal cannula.

    ____, ____, ____, ____

27. The echocardiogram indicates a large thrombus in the left atrium of a patient admitted with heart failure. During the night, the patient complains of severe, sudden onset left foot pain. You note that no pulse is palpable in the left foot and that it is cold and pale. Which action should you take next?
    1. Lower the patient's left foot below heart level.
    2. Administer oxygen at 4 L/minute to the patient.
    3. Notify the patient's physician about the assessment data.
    4. Check the patient's vital signs and oximetry.

28. A long-term-care resident with venous stasis ulcers is treated with Unna's boot. Which of the nursing activities included in the resident's care is best for you to delegate to a nursing assistant?
    1. Monitor capillary perfusion once every 8 hours.
    2. Teach family members the signs of infection.
    3. Evaluate foot sensation and movement each shift.
    4. Assist patient with cleaning around Unna's boot.

29. During the initial post-operative assessment of a patient who has just transferred to the post-anesthesia care unit (PACU) after repair of an abdominal aortic aneurysm, you obtain all of these data. Which has the most immediate implications for the patient's care?
    1. The arterial line indicates a blood pressure of 190/112.
    2. The monitor shows sinus rhythm with frequent PACs.
    3. The patient does not respond to verbal stimulation.
    4. The patient's urine output is 100 mL of amber urine.

30. As the manager of a cardiac surgery unit, you are responsible for developing a standardized care plan for the post-operative care of patients having cardiac surgery. Which of these nursing activities included in the care plan will need to be done by an RN?
    1. Remove chest and leg dressings on the second post-operative day and clean the incisions with antibacterial swabs.
    2. Reinforce patient and family teaching about the need to deep breathe and cough at least every 2 hours while awake.
    3. Develop individual plan for discharge teaching based on discharge medications and needed lifestyle changes.
    4. Administer oral analgesic medications as needed prior to assisting patient out of bed on first post-operative day.

CHAPTER 7

Hematologic Problems

1. You are reviewing the complete blood count (CBC) for a client who has been admitted for knee arthroscopy. Which value is most important to report to the physician prior to surgery?
   1. White blood cell count 16,000/mm³
   2. Hematocrit 33%
   3. Platelet count 426,000/mm³
   4. Hemoglobin 10.9 g/dL

2. A new RN is preparing to administer packed red blood cells (PRBCs) to a client whose anemia was caused by blood loss after surgery. Which action by the new RN requires that you, as charge nurse, intervene immediately?
   1. The new RN waits 20 minutes after obtaining the PRBCs before starting the infusion.
   2. The new RN starts an intravenous line for the transfusion using a 22-gauge catheter.
   3. The new RN primes the transfusion set using 5% dextrose in lactated Ringer's solution.
   4. The new RN tells the client that the PRBCs may cause a serious transfusion reaction.

3. A 32-year-old client with a history of sickle cell anemia is admitted to the hospital during a sickle cell crisis. The physician orders all of these interventions. Which order will you implement first?
   1. Give morphine sulfate 4–8 mg IV every hour as needed.
   2. Start a large-gauge IV line and infuse normal saline at 200 mL/hour.
   3. Immunize with Pneumovax and *Haemophilus influenzae* vaccines.
   4. Administer oxygen at an F_{IO_2} of 100% per non-rebreather mask.

4. A 78-year-old client admitted to the hospital with chronic anemia caused by possible gastrointestinal bleeding has all of these activities included in the care plan. Which activity is best delegated to an experienced nursing assistant (NA)?
   1. Use Hemoccult slides to obtain stool specimens.
   2. Have the client sign a colonoscopy consent form.
   3. Administer PEG-ES (GoLYTELY) bowel preparation.
   4. Check for allergies to contrast dye or shellfish.

5. As charge nurse, you are making the daily assignments on the medical-surgical unit. Which client is best assigned to a nurse who has floated from the post-anesthesia care unit (PACU)?
   1. A 30-year-old client with thalassemia major who has an order for subcutaneous infusion of deferoxamine (Desferal)
   2. A 43-year-old client with multiple myeloma who needs discharge teaching
   3. A 52-year-old client with chronic gastrointestinal bleeding who has returned to the unit after a colonoscopy
   4. A 65-year-old client with pernicious anemia who has just been admitted to the unit

6. You are making a room assignment for a newly arrived client whose laboratory testing indicates pancytopenia. All of these clients are already on the nursing unit. Which one will be the best roommate for the new client?
   1. The client with digoxin toxicity
   2. The client with viral pneumonia
   3. The client with shingles
   4. The client with cellulitis

7. A client admitted to the hospital with a sickle cell crisis complains of severe abdominal, hip, and knee pain. You observe an LPN accomplishing these client care tasks. Which one requires that you, as charge nurse, intervene immediately?
   1. The LPN encourages the client to use the ordered PCA.
   2. The LPN positions cold packs on the client's knees.
   3. The LPN places a "No Visitors" sign on the client's door.
   4. The LPN checks the client's temperature every 2 hours.

8. A 67-year-old client who is receiving chemotherapy for lung cancer is admitted to the hospital with thrombocytopenia. While you are taking the admission history, the client makes these statements. Which statement is of most concern?
   1. "I've noticed that I bruise more easily since the chemotherapy started."
   2. "My bowel movements are soft and dark brown in color."
   3. "I take one aspirin every morning because of my history of angina."
   4. "My appetite has decreased since the chemotherapy started."

9. Following a car accident, a client with a Medic-Alert bracelet indicating hemophilia A is admitted to the emergency department (ED). Which physician order should you implement first?
   1. Transport to radiology for C-spine x-rays.
   2. Transfuse Factor VII concentrate.
   3. Type and cross-match for 4 units RBCs.
   4. Infuse normal saline at 250 mL/hour.

10. As home health nurse, you are taking an admission history for a client who has a deep vein thrombosis and is taking warfarin (Coumadin) 2 mg daily. Which statement by the client is the best indicator that additional teaching about warfarin may be needed?
    1. "I have started to eat more healthy foods like green salads and fruit."
    2. "The doctor said that it is important to avoid becoming constipated."
    3. "Coumadin makes me feel a little nauseated unless I take it with food."
    4. "I will need to have some blood testing done once or twice a week."

11. A client is admitted to the intensive care unit (ICU) with disseminated intravascular coagulation (DIC) associated with a gram-negative infection. Which assessment information has the most immediate implications for the client's care?
    1. There is no palpable radial or pedal pulse.
    2. The client complains of chest pain.
    3. The client's oxygen saturation is 87%.
    4. There is mottling of the hands and feet.

12. A 22-year-old with stage I Hodgkin's disease is admitted to the oncology unit for radiation therapy. During the initial assessment, the client tells you, "Sometimes I am afraid of dying." Which response is most appropriate at this time?
    1. "Many individuals with this diagnosis have some fears."
    2. "Perhaps you should ask the doctor about medication."
    3. "Tell me a little bit more about your fear of dying."
    4. "Most people with stage I Hodgkin's disease survive."

13. After receiving change-of-shift report about all of these clients, which one will you assess first?
    1. A 26-year-old with thalassemia major who has a short-stay admission for a blood transfusion
    2. A 44-year-old who was admitted 3 days previously with a sickle cell crisis and has orders for a CT scan
    3. A 50-year-old with newly diagnosed stage IV non-Hodgkin's lymphoma who is crying and stating "I'm not ready to die"
    4. A 69-year-old with chemotherapy-induced neutropenia who has an elevated oral temperature

14. A long-term-care client with chronic lymphocytic leukemia has a nursing diagnosis of Activity Intolerance related to weakness and anemia. Which of these nursing activities is most appropriate for you, as the charge nurse, to delegate to a nursing assistant?
    1. Evaluate the client's response to normal activities of daily living.
    2. Check the client's blood pressure and pulse rate after ambulation.
    3. Determine which self-care activities the client can do independently.
    4. Assist the client in choosing a diet that will improve strength.

15. A transfusion of PRBCs has been infusing for 5 minutes when the client becomes flushed and tachypneic and says, "I am having chills. Please get me a blanket." Which action should you take first?
    1. Obtain a warm blanket for the client.
    2. Check the client's oral temperature.
    3. Stop the transfusion.
    4. Administer oxygen.

16. A group of clients is assigned to an RN–LPN/LVN team. The LPN/LVN is most likely to be assigned to provide client care and administer medications to which of these clients?
    1. A 36-year-old client with chronic renal failure who will need a subcutaneous injection of epoetin (Procrit)
    2. A 39-year-old client with hemophilia B who has been admitted for a blood transfusion
    3. A 50-year-old client with newly diagnosed polycythemia vera who is scheduled for phlebotomy
    4. A 55-year-old client with a history of stem cell transplantation who will have a bone marrow aspiration

17. You obtain the following data about a client admitted with multiple myeloma. Which information has the most immediate implications for the client's care?
    1. The client complains of chronic bone pain.
    2. The blood uric acid level is very elevated.
    3. The 24-hour urine shows Bence-Jones protein.
    4. The client is unable to plantarflex the feet.

18. The nurse in the outpatient clinic is assessing a 22-year-old with a history of a recent splenectomy after a motor vehicle accident. Which information obtained during the assessment will be of most immediate concern to the nurse?
    1. The client engages in unprotected sex.
    2. The client has an oral temperature of 99.7°F.
    3. The client has abdominal pain with light palpation.
    4. The client admits to occasional marijuana use.

19. A client with graft-versus-host disease (GVHD) after a bone marrow transplant is being cared for on the medical unit. Which of these nursing activities is best delegated to a newly graduated RN who has had a 6-week orientation to the unit?
    1. Administration of methotrexate and cyclosporine to the client
    2. Assessment of the client for signs of infection caused by GVHD
    3. Infusion of D_5.45% normal saline at 125 mL/hour to the client
    4. Education of the client about ways to prevent infection

20. You are the charge nurse in an oncology unit. A client with an absolute neutrophil count (ANC) of 300/mm³ is placed in protective isolation. Which staff member should you assign to provide care for this client, under the supervision of an experienced oncology RN?
    1. An LPN who has floated from the same-day-surgery unit
    2. An RN from the float pool who usually works on the surgical unit
    3. An LPN with 2 years of experience on the oncology unit
    4. An RN who transferred recently from the ED

21. You are transferring a client with newly diagnosed chronic myeloid leukemia to a long-term-care (LTC) facility. Which information is most important to communicate to the LTC charge nurse prior to transferring the client?
    1. The Philadelphia chromosome is present in the blood smear.
    2. Glucose is elevated as a result of prednisone therapy.
    3. There has been a 20-pound weight loss over the last year.
    4. The client's chemotherapy has resulted in neutropenia.

22. A client with acute myelogenous leukemia is receiving induction phase chemotherapy. Which assessment information is of most concern?
    1. Serum potassium level of 7.8 mEq/L
    2. Urine output less than intake by 400 mL
    3. Inflammation and redness of oral mucosa
    4. Ecchymoses present on anterior trunk

23. A client who has been receiving cyclosporine following an organ transplant is experiencing these symptoms. Which one is of most concern?
    1. Bleeding of the gums while brushing the teeth
    2. Non-tender swelling in the right groin
    3. Occasional nausea after taking the medication
    4. Numbness and tingling of the feet

24. You have developed the nursing diagnosis Risk for Impaired Tissue Integrity related to effects of radiation for a client with Hodgkin's lymphoma who is receiving radiation to the groin area. Which nursing activity is best delegated to a nursing assistant caring for the client?
    1. Check the skin for signs of redness or peeling.
    2. Apply alcohol-free lotion to the area after cleaning.
    3. Explain good skin care to the client and family.
    4. Clean the skin over the area daily with a mild soap.

25. After receiving the change-of-shift report, which client will you assess first?
    1. A 20-year-old with possible acute myelogenous leukemia who has just arrived on the medical unit
    2. A 38-year-old with aplastic anemia who needs teaching about decreasing infection risk prior to discharge
    3. A 40-year-old with lymphedema who requests help to put on compression stockings before getting out of bed
    4. A 60-year-old with non-Hodgkin's lymphoma who is refusing the ordered chemotherapy regimen

CHAPTER 8

Neurologic Problems

1. What is the priority nursing diagnosis for a patient experiencing a migraine headache?
   1. Acute Pain related to biologic and chemical factors
   2. Anxiety related to change in or threat to health status
   3. Hopelessness related to deteriorating physiological condition
   4. Risk for Side Effects related to medical therapy

2. You are creating a teaching plan for a patient with newly diagnosed migraine headaches. Which key items should be included in the teaching plan? (Choose all that apply.)
   1. Avoid foods that contain tyramine, such as alcohol and aged cheese.
   2. Avoid drugs such as Tagamet, nitroglycerin, and nifedipine.
   3. Abortive therapy is aimed at eliminating the pain during the aura.
   4. A potential side effect of medications is rebound headache.
   5. Complementary therapies such as relaxation may be helpful.
   6. Continue taking estrogen as prescribed by your physician.

3. The patient with migraine headaches has a seizure. After the seizure, which action can you delegate to the nursing assistant?
   1. Document the seizure.
   2. Perform neurologic checks.
   3. Take the patient's vital signs.
   4. Restrain the patient for protection.

4. You are preparing to admit a patient with a seizure disorder. Which of the following actions can you delegate to the LPN/LVN?
   1. Complete admission assessment.
   2. Set up oxygen and suction equipment.
   3. Place a padded tongue blade at bedside.
   4. Pad the side rails before patient arrives.

5. A nursing student is teaching a patient and family about epilepsy prior to the patient's discharge. For which statement should you intervene?
   1. "You should avoid consumption of all forms of alcohol."
   2. "Wear your medical alert bracelet at all times."
   3. "Protect your loved one's airway during a seizure."
   4. "It's OK to take over-the-counter medications."

6. A patient with Parkinson's disease has a nursing diagnosis of Impaired Physical Mobility related to neuromuscular impairment. You observe a nursing assistant performing all of these actions. For which action must you intervene?
   1. The NA assists the patient to ambulate to the bathroom and back to bed.
   2. The NA reminds the patient not to look at his feet when he is walking.
   3. The NA performs the patient's complete bath and oral care.
   4. The NA sets up the patient's tray and encourages patient to feed himself.

7. The nurse is preparing to discharge a patient with chronic low back pain. Which statement by the patient indicates that additional teaching is necessary?
   1. "I will avoid exercise because the pain gets worse."
   2. "I will use heat or ice to help control the pain."
   3. "I will not wear high-heeled shoes at home or work."
   4. "I will purchase a firm mattress to replace my old one."

8. A patient with a spinal cord injury (SCI) complains about a severe throbbing headache that suddenly started a short time ago. Assessment of the patient reveals increased blood pressure (168/94) and decreased heart rate (48/minute), diaphoreses, and flushing of the face and neck. What action should you take first?
   1. Administer the ordered acetaminophen (Tylenol).
   2. Check the Foley tubing for kinks or obstruction.
   3. Adjust the temperature in the patient's room.
   4. Notify the physician about the change in status.

9. Which patient should you, as charge nurse, assign to a new graduate RN who is orienting to the neurologic unit?
   1. A 28-year-old newly admitted patient with spinal cord injury
   2. A 67-year-old patient with stroke 3 days ago and left-sided weakness
   3. A 85-year-old dementia patient to be transferred to long-term care today
   4. A 54-year-old patient with Parkinson's who needs assistance with bathing

10. A patient with a spinal cord injury at level C3-4 is being cared for in the ED. What is the priority assessment?
    1. Determine the level at which the patient has intact sensation.
    2. Assess the level at which the patient has retained mobility.
    3. Check blood pressure and pulse for signs of spinal shock.
    4. Monitor respiratory effort and oxygen saturation level.

11. You are pulled from the ED to the neurologic floor. Which action should you delegate to the nursing assistant when providing nursing care for a patient with SCI?
    1. Assess patient's respiratory status every 4 hours.
    2. Take patient's vital signs and record every 4 hours.
    3. Monitor nutritional status including calorie counts.
    4. Have patient turn, cough, and deep breathe every 2 hours.

12. You are helping the patient with an SCI to establish a bladder-retraining program. What strategies may stimulate the patient to void? (Choose all that apply.)
    1. Stroke the patient's inner thigh.
    2. Pull on the patient's pubic hair.
    3. Initiate intermittent straight catheterization.
    4. Pour warm water over the perineum.
    5. Tap the bladder to stimulate detrusor muscle.

13. The patient with a cervical SCI has been placed in fixed skeletal traction with a halo fixation device. When caring for this patient the nurse may delegate which action(s) to the LPN/LVN? (Choose all that apply.)
    1. Check the patient's skin for pressure from device.
    2. Assess the patient's neurologic status for changes.
    3. Observe the halo insertion sites for signs of infection.
    4. Clean the halo insertion sites with hydrogen peroxide.

14. You are preparing a nursing care plan for the patient with SCI including the nursing diagnoses Impaired Physical Mobility and Self-Care Deficit. The patient tells you, "I don't know why we're doing all this. My life's over." What additional nursing diagnosis takes priority based on this statement?
    1. Risk for Injury related to altered mobility
    2. Imbalanced Nutrition, Less Than Body Requirements
    3. Impaired Adjustment to Spinal Cord Injury
    4. Poor Body Image related to immobilization

15. Which patient should be assigned to the traveling nurse, new to neurologic nursing care, who has been on the neurologic unit for 1 week?
    1. A 34-year-old patient newly diagnosed with multiple sclerosis (MS)
    2. A 68-year-old patient with chronic amyotrophic lateral sclerosis (ALS)
    3. A 56-year-old patient with Guillain-Barré syndrome (GBS) in respiratory distress
    4. A 25-year-old patient admitted with C4 level spinal cord injury (SCI)

16. The patient with multiple sclerosis tells the nursing assistant that after physical therapy she is too tired to take a bath. What is your priority nursing diagnosis at this time?
    1. Fatigue related to disease state
    2. Activity Intolerance due to generalized weakness
    3. Impaired Physical Mobility related to neuromuscular impairment
    4. Self-care Deficit related to fatigue and neuromuscular weakness

17. The LPN/LVN, under your supervision, is providing nursing care for a patient with GBS. What observation would you instruct the LPN/LVN to report immediately?
    1. Complaints of numbness and tingling
    2. Facial weakness and difficulty speaking
    3. Rapid heart rate of 102 beats per minute
    4. Shallow respirations and decreased breath sounds

18. The nursing assistant reports to you, the RN, that the patient with myasthenia gravis (MG) has an elevated temperature (102.2°F), heart rate of 120/minute, rise in blood pressure (158/94), and was incontinent of urine and stool. What is your best first action at this time?
    1. Administer an acetaminophen suppository.
    2. Notify the physician immediately.
    3. Recheck vital signs in 1 hour.
    4. Reschedule patient's physical therapy.

19. You are providing care for a patient with an acute hemorrhagic stroke. The patient's husband has been reading a lot about strokes and asks why his wife did not receive alteplase. What is your best response?
    1. "Your wife was not admitted within the time frame that alteplase is usually given."
    2. "This drug is used primarily for patients who experience an acute heart attack."
    3. "Alteplase dissolves clots and may cause more bleeding into your wife's brain."
    4. "Your wife had gallbladder surgery just 6 months ago and this prevents the use of alteplase."

20. You are supervising a senior nursing student who is caring for a patient with a right hemisphere stroke. Which action by the student nurse requires that you intervene?
    1. The student instructs the patient to sit up straight, resulting in the patient's puzzled expression.
    2. The student moves the patient's tray to the right side of her over-bed tray.
    3. The student assists the patient with passive range-of-motion (ROM) exercises.
    4. The student combs the left side of the patient's hair when the patient combs only the right side.

21. Which action(s) should you delegate to the experienced nursing assistant when caring for a patient with a thrombotic stroke with residual left-sided weakness? (Choose all that apply.)
    1. Assist patient to reposition every 2 hours.
    2. Reapply pneumatic compression boots.
    3. Remind patient to perform active ROM.
    4. Check extremities for redness and edema.

22. The patient who had a stroke needs to be fed. What instruction should you give to the nursing assistant who will feed the patient?
    1. Position the patient sitting up in bed before you feed her.
    2. Check the patient's gag and swallowing reflexes.
    3. Feed the patient quickly because there are three more waiting.
    4. Suction the patient's secretions between bites of food.

23. You have just admitted a patient with bacterial meningitis to the medical-surgical unit. The patient complains of a severe headache with photophobia and has a temperature of 102.6°F orally. Which collaborative intervention must be accomplished first?
    1. Administer codeine 15 mg orally for the patient's headache.
    2. Infuse ceftriaxone (Rocephin) 2000 mg IV to treat the infection.
    3. Give acetaminophen (Tylenol) 650 mg orally to reduce the fever.
    4. Give furosemide (Lasix) 40 mg IV to decrease intracranial pressure.

24. You are mentoring a student nurse in the intensive care unit (ICU) while caring for a patient with meningococcal meningitis. Which action by the student requires that you intervene immediately?
    1. The student enters the room without putting on a mask and gown.
    2. The student instructs the family that visits are restricted to 10 minutes.
    3. The student gives the patient a warm blanket when he says he feels cold.
    4. The student checks the patient's pupil response to light every 30 minutes.

25. A 23-year-old patient with a recent history of encephalitis is admitted to the medical unit with new-onset generalized tonic-clonic seizures. Which nursing activities included in the patient's care will be best to delegate to an LPN/LVN whom you are supervising? (Choose all that apply.)
    1. Document the onset time, nature of seizure activity, and postictal behaviors for all seizures.
    2. Administer phenytoin (Dilantin) 200 mg PO daily.
    3. Teach patient about the need for good oral hygiene.
    4. Develop a discharge plan, including physician visits and referral to the Epilepsy Foundation.

26. While working in the ICU, you are assigned to care for a patient with a seizure disorder. Which of these nursing actions will you implement first if the patient has a seizure?
    1. Place the patient on a non-rebreather mask with the oxygen at 15 L/minute.
    2. Administer lorazepam (Ativan) 1 mg IV.
    3. Turn the patient to the side and protect airway.
    4. Assess level of consciousness during and immediately after the seizure.

27. A patient recently started on phenytoin (Dilantin) to control simple complex seizures is seen in the outpatient clinic. Which information obtained during his chart review and assessment will be of greatest concern?
    1. The gums appear enlarged and inflamed.
    2. The white blood cell count is 2300/mm^3.
    3. Patient occasionally forgets to take the phenytoin until after lunch.
    4. Patient wants to renew his driver's license in the next month.

28. After receiving a change-of-shift report at 7:00 AM, which of these patients will you assess first?
    1. A 23-year-old with a migraine headache who is complaining of severe nausea associated with retching
    2. A 45-year-old who is scheduled for a craniotomy in 30 minutes and needs preoperative teaching
    3. A 59-year-old with Parkinson's disease who will need a swallowing assessment before breakfast
    4. A 63-year-old with multiple sclerosis who has an oral temperature of 101.8°F and flank pain

29. All of these nursing activities are included in the care plan for a 78-year-old man with Parkinson's disease who has been referred to your home health agency. Which ones will you delegate to a nursing assistant (NA)? (Choose all that apply.)
    1. Check for orthostatic changes in pulse and blood pressure.
    2. Monitor for improvement in tremor after levodopa (L-dopa) is given.
    3. Remind the patient to allow adequate time for meals.
    4. Monitor for abnormal involuntary jerky movements of extremities.
    5. Assist the patient with prescribed strengthening exercises.
    6. Adapt the patient's preferred activities to his level of function.

30. As the manger in a long-term-care (LTC) facility, you are in charge of developing a standard plan of care for residents with Alzheimer's disease. Which of these nursing tasks is best to delegate to the LPN team leaders working in the facility?
    1. Check for improvement in resident memory after medication therapy is initiated.
    2. Use the Mini-Mental State Examination to assess residents every 6 months.
    3. Assist residents to toilet every 2 hours to decrease risk for urinary incontinence.
    4. Develop individualized activity plans after consulting with residents and family.

31. A patient who has been admitted to the medical unit with new-onset angina also has a diagnosis of Alzheimer's disease. Her husband tells you that he rarely gets a good night's sleep because he needs to be sure she does not wander during the night. He insists on checking each of the medications you give her to be sure they are the same as the ones she takes at home. Based on this information, which nursing diagnosis is most appropriate for this patient?
    1. Decreased Cardiac Output related to poor myocardial contractility
    2. Caregiver Role Strain related to continuous need for providing care
    3. Ineffective Therapeutic Regimen Management related to poor patient memory
    4. Risk for Falls related to patient wandering behavior during the night

32. You are caring for a patient with a recurrent glioblastoma who is receiving dexamethasone (Decadron) 4 mg IV every 6 hours to relieve symptoms of right arm weakness and headache. Which assessment information concerns you the most?
    1. The patient does not recognize family members.
    2. The blood glucose level is 234 mg/dL.
    3. The patient complains of a continued headache.
    4. The daily weight has increased 1 kg.

33. A 70-year-old alcoholic patient with acute lethargy, confusion, and incontinence is admitted to the hospital ED. His wife tells you that he fell down the stairs about a month ago, but "he didn't have a scratch afterward." She feels that he has become gradually less active and sleepier over the last 10 days or so. Which of the following collaborative interventions will you implement first?
    1. Place on the hospital alcohol withdrawal protocol.
    2. Transfer to radiology for a CT scan.
    3. Insert a retention catheter to straight drainage.
    4. Give phenytoin (Dilantin) 100 mg PO.

34. Which of these patients in the neurologic ICU will be best to assign to an RN who has floated from the medical unit?
    1. A 26-year-old patient with a basilar skull fracture who has clear drainage coming out of the nose
    2. A 42-year-old patient admitted several hours ago with a headache and diagnosed with a ruptured berry aneurysm
    3. A 46-year-old patient who was admitted 48 hours ago with bacterial meningitis and has an antibiotic dose due
    4. A 65-year-old patient with an astrocytoma who has just returned to the unit after having a craniotomy

CHAPTER 9

Visual and Auditory Problems

1. You are working in an ambulatory clinic. A client calls to report redness to the sclera, itching of the eyes and increased lacrimation for several hours. What should you direct the caller to do first?
   1. "Please call your doctor." (Refuse to advise.)
   2. "Apply a cool compress to your eyes."
   3. "If you are wearing contact lenses, remove them."
   4. "Take an over-the-counter antihistamine."

2. You are teaching prevention of accidental eye injuries in a community health clinic to a church group. What is the most important thing to stress?
   1. Follow workplace policies for handling chemicals.
   2. Children and parents should be cautious about aggressive play.
   3. Wear protective eyewear during sports or hazardous work.
   4. Establish emergency eyewash stations in the workplace.

3. Which client(s) would be best to assign to an experienced nurse in an ambulatory eye surgery center? (Choose all that apply.)
   1. A client who needs post-operative instructions for cataract surgery
   2. A client who needs an eye-pad and a metal shield applied
   3. A client who needs home health referral for dressing changes and eye drops
   4. A client who needs teaching about self-administration of eye drops

4. Place these steps for eye drop administration in the correct order.
   1. Gently press on the lacrimal duct for 1 minute.
   2. Gently pull downward to expose the lower conjunctival sac.
   3. Have the client gently close the eye and move it around.
   4. Have the client look up while you instill the number of prescribed drops.
   5. Hold the dropper and stabilize your hand on the client's forehead.
   6. Have the client sit down with head slightly hyperextended.

   ____, ____, ____, ____, ____, ____

5. Which of these tasks are appropriate to delegate to the LPN/LVN who is functioning under the supervision of an RN? (Choose all that apply.)
   1. Assess the sexual implications for a client with oculogenital type *Chlamydia trachomatis*.
   2. Administer sulfacetamide sodium 10% (Sulf-10 Ophthalmic) to a child with conjunctivitis.
   3. Review handwashing and hygiene practices with clients who have eye infections.
   4. Show clients how to gently cleanse eyelid margins to remove crusting.

6. An excited mother calls you for advice. "My child got cleaning solution in the eyes and I rinsed it out with water. What should I do? She is still screaming!" What do you instruct the caller to do immediately?
   1. Comfort the child and check vision.
   2. Continue to irrigate eyes with water.
   3. Call Poison Control.
   4. Call 911.

7. You are working in a community health clinic and a client needs instructions for care of a hordeolum (sty) to the right upper eyelid. What is the first treatment that the client should try?
   1. Apply warm compresses 4 times/day.
   2. Gently perform hygienic eyelid scrubs.
   3. Obtain prescription for antibiotic drops.
   4. Contact the ophthalmologist.

8. Which of the following should be immediately reported to the physician?
   1. Change in color vision
   2. Crusty yellow drainage on eyelashes
   3. Increased lacrimation
   4. Curtain-like shadow across visual field

9. For a client who has sustained recent blindness, which task(s) would be appropriate to delegate to the nursing assistant? (Choose all that apply.)
   1. Listen to the client express grief or loss.
   2. Assist client to ambulate in hall.
   3. Orient client to surroundings.
   4. Encourage independence.

10. In discharge teaching for cataract surgery, the client and family should be told to immediately report which symptom to the physician?
    1. Scratchy sensation in the operative eye
    2. Loss of depth perception with the patch in place
    3. Inadequate vision 6–8 hours after the patch is removed
    4. Intense pain not relieved by prescribed medications

11. Glaucoma is a preventable condition. Which group is most likely to develop glaucoma and should be targeted for educational programs?
    1. African-Americans of any age
    2. Alaskan-Americans >50 years
    3. White-Americans >60 years
    4. Native-Americans >35 years

12. Before giving a beta-adrenergic blocker glaucoma agent, you would notify the physician if the client discloses a history of what condition?
    1. Hypertension
    2. Tachycardia
    3. Rheumatoid arthritis
    4. Bradycardia

13. Which of these tasks are appropriate to delegate to the LPN/LVN who is functioning under the supervision of a team leader or RN? (Choose all that apply.)
    1. Irrigate the ear canal for impacted cerumen.
    2. Administer amoxicillin to a child with otitis media.
    3. Remind the client not to blow nose after tympanoplasty.
    4. Counsel the client with Ménière's disease.

14. You are reviewing the drug list of an elderly client who is on several medications prescribed by different specialists for various health problems. The client reports "lately there has been a roaring sound in my ears." You notify the prescriber of which medication?
    1. gentamicin sulfate (Garamycin)
    2. metoprolol (Lopressor)
    3. amoxicillin (Amoxil)
    4. warfarin (Coumadin)

15. A cheerful, elderly widow comes to the community clinic for her annual check-up. She is in reasonably good health, but she has a hearing loss of 40 dB. She confides, "I don't get out much. I used to be really active, but the older I get, the more trouble I have hearing. It can be really embarrassing." What is the priority nursing diagnosis?
    1. Social Interaction, Impaired related to perceived inability to interact
    2. Disturbed Sensory Perception related to progressive hearing loss
    3. Knowledge Deficit related to pathophysiological processes
    4. Coping, Ineffective related to change in sensory abilities

16. Which physical assessment finding should be reported to the physician?
    1. Pearly gray or pink tympanic membrane
    2. Dense, whitish ring at the circumference of the tympanum
    3. Bulging red or blue tympanic membrane
    4. A cone of light at the innermost part of the tympanum

17. You are taking histories from several clients who report vertigo. Which client report concerns you the most?
    1. Vertigo with hearing loss
    2. Episodic vertigo
    3. Vertigo without hearing loss
    4. "Merry-go-round" vertigo

18. In assisting clients with vertigo and balance problems, which team members (RN, LPN/LVN, MD, physical therapist, nursing assistant), working under appropriate supervision, should be assigned to fulfill each task?

    1. Assess and identify the etiology of vertigo. _____

    2. Assist the client in routine position change and ambulation. _____

    3. Administer antivertigo agents, such as meclizine (Antivert). _____

    4. Obtain informed consent for a labyrinthectomy. _____

    5. Assess situations that lead to or exacerbate vertigo._____

19. You are reviewing your client's understanding of the post-operative stapedectomy instructions that you gave several days ago. Which comment concerns you the most?
    1. "I'm going to take swimming lessons in a couple of months."
    2. "I have to take a long overseas flight in several weeks."
    3. "I can't wait to get back to my regular weightlifting class."
    4. "I have been coughing a lot with my mouth open."

20. Place the steps for removal of a foreign body from the ear canal in the correct order.
    1. Refer for treatment of external otitis.
    2. Inspect the tympanic membrane for trauma.
    3. Obtain history for type of object.
    4. Choose appropriate fluid for irrigation or instillation.
    5. Assess for possibility of perforation.

    _____, _____, _____, _____, _____

CHAPTER 10

Musculoskeletal Problems

1. You are initiating a nursing care plan for a patient with osteoporosis. All of these nursing interventions apply to the nursing diagnosis Risk for Falls. Which intervention should you delegate to the nursing assistant?
   1. Identify environmental factors that increase risk for falls.
   2. Monitor gait, balance, and fatigue level with ambulation.
   3. Collaborate with physical therapy to provide patient with walker.
   4. Assist the patient with ambulation to bathroom and in halls.

2. You are preparing to teach a newly diagnosed patient with osteoporosis about strategies to prevent falls. Which of these points will you be sure to include? (Choose all that apply.)
   1. Wear a hip protector when ambulating.
   2. Remove throw rugs and other obstacles at home.
   3. Exercise will help build your strength.
   4. You should expect a few bumps and bruises when you go home.
   5. When you are tired, you should rest.

3. You discover all of these assessment findings when admitting a patient with Paget's disease. Which finding indicates that the physician should be notified?
   1. The patient has bowing of both legs and the knees are asymmetric.
   2. The base of the patient's skull is invaginated (platybasia).
   3. The patient is only 5 feet tall and weighs 120 pounds.
   4. The patient's skull is soft, thick, and larger than normal.

4. As charge nurse you observe the LPN/LVN providing all of these interventions for the patient with Paget's disease. Which action requires that you intervene?
   1. Administers 600 mg of ibuprofen to the patient
   2. Encourages the patient to perform PT recommended exercises
   3. Applies ice and gentle massage to the patient's lower extremities
   4. Reminds the patient to drink milk and eat cottage cheese

5. As charge nurse you are making assignments for the day shift. Which patient would you assign to the nurse who has been pulled from the post-anesthesia care unit (PACU) for the day?
   1. A 35-year-old patient with osteomyelitis who needs teaching prior to hyperbaric oxygen therapy
   2. A 62-year-old patient with osteomalacia who is being discharged to a long-term care facility
   3. A 68-year-old patient with osteoporosis and a new orthotic device whose knowledge of use of this device must be assessed
   4. A 72-year-old patient with Paget's disease who has just returned from surgery for total knee replacement

6. You delegate taking vital signs to an experienced nursing assistant. The patient has been diagnosed with osteomyelitis. Which vital sign do you want the nursing assistant to report immediately?
   1. Temperature 99.9°F
   2. Blood pressure 136/80
   3. Heart rate 96/minute
   4. Respiratory rate 24/minute

7. You are working with a nursing assistant to provide care for six patients. At the beginning of the shift, you carefully tell the nursing assistant what patient interventions and tasks she will be expected to perform. To be sure that your communication is appropriate, you refer to the 4 C's. List the 4 C's below.

   _____

   _____

   _____

   _____

8. You are providing nursing care for a patient with carpal tunnel syndrome (CTS) who is preparing for surgery. Which intervention should you delegate to the nursing assistant?
   1. Initiate placement of a splint for immobilization during the day.
   2. Assess the patient's wrist and hand for discoloration and brittle nails.
   3. Assist the patient with daily self-care measures such as bathing and eating.
   4. Test the patient for painful tingling in the four digits of the hand.

9. You observe the nursing assistant performing all of these interventions for the patient with CTS. Which action requires that you intervene immediately?
   1. Arrange the patient's lunch tray and cut the meat.
   2. Provide warm water and assist the patient with a bath.
   3. Replace the patient's splint in hyperextension position.
   4. Remind the patient not to lift very heavy objects.

10. The patient is scheduled for endoscopic carpal tunnel release surgery in the morning. What key point will you be sure to teach the patient?
    1. Pain and numbness will be experienced for several days to weeks.
    2. Immediately after surgery, the patient will no longer need assistance.
    3. After surgery, the dressing will be large with lots of drainage.
    4. After surgery, the pain and paresthesia will no longer be present.

11. As charge nurse you assign the nursing care of a patient who has just returned from open carpal tunnel release surgery to an experienced LPN/LVN, who will perform under the supervision of an RN. Which of the following instructions will you provide for the LPN/LVN? (Choose all that apply.)
    1. Check the patient's vital signs every 15 minutes in the first hour.
    2. Check the dressing for drainage and tightness.
    3. Elevate the patient's hand above the heart.
    4. The patient will no longer need pain medication.
    5. Check the neurovascular status of the fingers every hour.

12. You are preparing the post-operative CTS patient for discharge. Which information is important to provide to this patient?
    1. The surgical procedure is a cure for CTS.
    2. Hand movements will be restricted for 4–6 weeks after surgery.
    3. Frequent pain medication dosages will no longer be necessary.
    4. Notify the physician immediately for any pain or discomfort.

13. During discharge preparations, a patient with osteoporosis makes all of these statements. Which statement indicates to you that the patient needs additional teaching?
    1. "I take my ibuprofen every morning as soon as I get up."
    2. "My daughter removed all of the throw rugs in my home."
    3. "My husband helps me every afternoon with range-of-motion exercises."
    4. "I rest in my recliner chair every day for at least an hour."

14. The patient suffered a fractured femur. Which of the following would you tell the nursing assistant to report immediately?
    1. The patient complains of pain.
    2. The patient appears confused.
    3. The patient's blood pressure is 136/88.
    4. The patient voided using the bedpan.

15. After change-of-shift report, which patient should the nurse assess first?
    1. A 42-year-old patient with carpal tunnel syndrome complaining of pain
    2. A 64-year-old patient with osteoporosis who is waiting for discharge
    3. A 28-year-old patient with fracture complaining that the cast is tight
    4. A 56-year-old patient with left leg amputation complaining of phantom pain

16. A patient with a fractured fibula is receiving skeletal traction and has skeletal pins in place. You instruct the nursing assistant to immediately report which of the following?
    1. The patient wants to change position in bed.
    2. There is a small amount of clear fluid on the pin sites.
    3. The traction weights are resting on the floor.
    4. The patient is complaining of pain and muscle spasm.

17. A patient with a fracture of the right ankle has a nursing diagnosis of Impaired Physical Mobility. As charge nurse you observe a new graduate RN perform all of these interventions. For which action should you intervene?
    1. Encourages the patient to go from lying to standing position
    2. Administers pain medication prior to beginning exercises
    3. Explains to the patient and family the purpose of the exercise program
    4. Reminds the patient about correct usage of crutches

18. The charge nurse assigns the nursing care of a patient who is 1 day post-operative after a left below-the-knee amputation to an experienced LPN/LVN, who will function under your supervision. When you instruct the LPN/LVN, what will you describe as the major focus for care today?
    1. To attain pain control for phantom pain.
    2. To monitor for signs of sufficient tissue perfusion.
    3. To assist the patient to ambulate as soon as possible.
    4. To elevate the residual limb when the patient is supine.

19. A patient with a right above-the-knee amputation has phantom limb pain (PLP) and asks you why. What is your best response?
    1. "Phantom limb pain is not explained or predicted by any one theory."
    2. "Phantom limb pain occurs because your body thinks your leg is still present. "
    3. "Phantom limb pain will not interfere with your activities of daily living."
    4. "Phantom limb pain is not real pain, but is remembered pain."

20. During morning care, the patient with a below-the-knee amputation asks the nursing assistant about prostheses. How should you instruct the nursing assistant to respond?
    1. "You should get a prosthesis so that you can walk again."
    2. "Wait and ask your doctor that question next time he comes in."
    3. "It's too soon to be worrying about getting a prosthesis."
    4. "I'll ask the nurse to come in and discuss this with you."

21. During assessment of a patient with fractures of the medial ulna and radius, you find all of the following data. Which assessment finding should you report to the physician immediately?
    1. The patient complains of pressure and pain.
    2. The cast is in place and is dry and intact.
    3. The skin is pink and warm to touch.
    4. The patient can move all fingers and thumb.

CHAPTER 11

Gastrointestinal and Nutritional Problems

1. In preparing a client for a colonoscopy procedure, which task is most suitable to delegate to the nursing assistant?
   1. Explain the need for clear liquids 1–3 days prior to procedure.
   2. Reinforce NPO status 8 hours prior to procedure.
   3. Administer laxatives 1–3 days prior to procedure.
   4. Administer an enema the night before the procedure.

2. You would be most concerned about which client having an order for TPN (total parental nutrition) fat emulsion?
   1. A client with gastrointestinal obstruction
   2. A client with severe anorexia nervosa
   3. A client with chronic diarrhea and vomiting
   4. A client with a fractured femur

3. You are preparing to administer TPN through a central line. Place the steps for administration in the correct order.
   1. Use aseptic technique when handling the injection cap.
   2. Thread the IV tubing through an infusion pump.
   3. Check the solution for cloudiness or turbidity.
   4. Connect the tubing to the central line.
   5. Select the correct tubing and filter.
   6. Set infusion pump at prescribed rate.

   ____, ____, ____, ____, ____, ____

4. You are caring for a client with peptic ulcer disease. Which assessment finding is the most serious?
   1. Projectile vomiting
   2. Burning sensation 2 hours after eating
   3. Coffee-ground emesis
   4. Board-like abdomen with shoulder pain

5. You are taking an initial history for a client seeking surgical treatment for obesity. Which of the following should be called to the attention of the surgeon before proceeding with additional history or physical assessment?
   1. Obesity for approximately 5 years
   2. History of counseling for body dysmorphic disorder
   3. Failure to reduce weight with other forms of therapy
   4. Body weight 100% above the ideal for age, gender, and height

6. In educating a client with gastroesophageal reflux disease (GERD), you will teach the client that the drug therapy is a "step-up" approach that depends on the response to the medication. For the drugs listed, what is the anticipated order that the physician will try in the treatment plan?
   1. magnesium trisilicate (Gaviscon) and famotidine (Pepcid AC)
   2. ranitidine (Zantac) 150 mg
   3. pantoprazole (Protonix)

   _____, _____, _____

7. In caring for a client with GERD, which task would be appropriate to assign to the nursing assistant?
   1. Share successful strategies for weight reduction.
   2. Encourage the client to express concerns about lifestyle modification.
   3. Remind the client not to lie down for 2–3 hours after eating.
   4. Explain the rationale for small frequent meals.

8. You are preparing to give an enteral feeding through a nasogastric tube. Place the steps in the correct order.
   1. Assess for bowel sounds.
   2. Auscultate tube placement and check pH.
   3. Flush the tube with water.
   4. Reflush the tube with water.
   5. Administer the feeding.
   6. Check for residual volume.

   _____, _____, _____, _____, _____, _____

9. Care for which of these clients is most appropriate to assign to the LPN/LVN, under the supervision of an RN?
   1. A client with oral cancer who is scheduled in the morning for glossectomy
   2. An obese client returned from surgery following a vertical banded gastroplasty
   3. A client with anorexia nervosa with muscle weakness and decreased urine output
   4. A client with intractable nausea and vomiting related to chemotherapy

10. In planning the post-operative care for a morbidly obese client, how can the expertise of the LPN/LVN best be applied?
    1. Obtain an oversized blood pressure cuff and a large-size bed.
    2. Set up a reinforced trapeze bar.
    3. Assist in the planning of bathing, turning, and ambulation.
    4. Design alternatives for routine tasks such as daily weights.

11. A client with proctitis needs a rectal suppository. A senior nursing student assigned to this client tells you that she is afraid to insert the suppository because she has never done it before. What is the most appropriate action in supervising this student?
    1. You give the medication and report the student to the instructor.
    2. Ask the student to leave the clinical area for being unprepared.
    3. Reassign the client to an LPN/LVN.
    4. Show the student how to insert the suppository and talk to the instructor.

12. You are teaching the client and family how to do colostomy irrigation. Place the information in the correct order.
    1. Hang the container at about shoulder height.
    2. Allow the solution to flow slowly and steadily for 5–10 minutes.
    3. Put 500–1000 mL of lukewarm water in the container.
    4. Allow 30–45 minutes for evacuation.
    5. Lubricate the stoma cone and gently insert the tubing tip into the stoma.
    6. Clean, rinse, and dry skin, and apply a new drainage pouch.
    7. Put on a pair of clean gloves

    ____, ____, ____, ____, ____, ____, ____

13. You are caring for a client with a nasogastric (NG) tube. Which task can be delegated to the experienced nursing assistant?
    1. Remove the NG tube per physician order.
    2. Secure the tape if the client accidentally dislodges the tube.
    3. Disconnect the suction to allow ambulation to the toilet.
    4. Reconnect the suction after the client has ambulated.

14. In planning a treatment and prevention program of chronic fecal incontinence for an elderly client, which intervention should you try first?
    1. Administer a glycerin suppository 15 minutes before evacuation time.
    2. Insert a rectal tube at specified intervals each day.
    3. Assist the client to the bedpan or toilet 30 minutes after meals.
    4. Use incontinence briefs or adult-sized diapers.

15. A client hospitalized with ulcerative colitis reports 10–20 small diarrhea stools per day, with abdominal pain prior to defecation. The client appears depressed and underweight and is uninterested in self-care or suggested therapies. What is the priority nursing diagnosis?
    1. Diarrhea related to irritated bowel
    2. Imbalanced Nutrition: Less Than Body Requirements related to nutrient loss
    3. Acute Pain related to increased GI motility
    4. Ineffective Therapeutic Regimen related to treatment plan

16. While transferring a dirty laundry bag, a nursing assistant sustains a puncture wound to the finger from a contaminated needle. The unit has several clients with hepatitis and AIDS; the source is unknown. Prioritize the instructions that you, as charge nurse, should give to the assistant.
    1. Have blood test(s) drawn per protocol.
    2. Complete and file an incident report.
    3. Perform a thorough aseptic handwashing.
    4. Report to the occupational health nurse.
    5. Follow up for results and counseling.
    6. Begin prophylactic drug therapy.

    ____, ____, ____, ____, ____, ____

17. You are caring for an obese post-operative client who underwent surgery for bowel resection. As the client is moving in bed, he states, "Something popped open." Upon examination you note wound evisceration. Place the following steps in order for handling this complication.
    1. Cover the intestine with sterile moistened gauze.
    2. Stay calm and stay with the client.
    3. Monitor the vital signs, especially BP and pulse.
    4. Have a colleague gather supplies and contact the physician.
    5. Put the client into semi-Fowler's with knees slightly flexed.
    6. Prepare the client for surgery as ordered.

    ____, ____, ____, ____, ____, ____

18. You are caring for a post-operative cholecystectomy client. What should be reported immediately to the physician?
    1. The client cannot void 4 hours post-operatively.
    2. The client reports shoulder pain.
    3. The client reports severe RUQ tenderness.
    4. Output does not equal input for the first few hours.

19. In caring for a client with acute viral hepatitis, which task should be delegated to the nursing assistant?
    1. Empty the bedpan while wearing gloves.
    2. Suggest diversional activities.
    3. Monitor dietary preferences.
    4. Report signs and symptoms of jaundice.

20. A client with cirrhosis is at risk for developing complications. Which condition is the most serious and potentially life-threatening?
    1. Esophageal varices
    2. Ascites
    3. Peripheral edema
    4. Asterixis (liver flap)

21. For clients coming to the ambulatory care GI clinic, which task would be most appropriate to assign to the LPN/LVN?
    1. Teach a client self-care measures for hemorrhoids.
    2. Assist the physician in incision and drainage of a pilonidal cyst.
    3. Evaluate a client's response to sitz baths for an anorectal abscess.
    4. Describe the basic pathophysiology of an anal fistula to a client.

22. A client underwent an exploratory laparotomy 2 days ago. The physician should be called immediately for which physical assessment finding?
    1. Abdominal distention and rigidity
    2. NG tube intentionally displaced by client
    3. Absent or hypoactive bowel sounds
    4. Nausea and occasional vomiting

23. You must rearrange the room assignment for several clients. Which two clients would be best suited to put in the same room?
    1. A 35-year old female with copious, intractable diarrhea and vomiting
    2. A 43-year old female second day post-operative cholecystectomy
    3. A 53-year old female with pain related to alcohol-associated pancreatitis
    4. A 62-year old female with colon cancer receiving chemotherapy and radiation

    _____ , _____

24. As nurse manager, you must select an employee to participate in a hospital committee that will develop client education brochures about common abdominal surgeries and wound care. Who would be the best employee to send to this committee?
    1. Newly graduated medical-surgical RN
    2. Experienced medical-surgical RN
    3. Experienced surgical intensive care unit RN
    4. Experienced medical-surgical LPN/LVN

25. A client is admitted through the emergency department for a strangulated intestinal obstruction with perforation. What interventions do you anticipate for this emergency condition? (Choose all that apply.)
    1. Preparation for surgery
    2. Barium enema
    3. NG tube insertion
    4. Abdominal x-ray
    5. IV fluids

26. Place the steps in correct order for performing colostomy care.
    1. Fit the pouch snugly around the stoma.
    2. Assess the color and appearance of the stoma.
    3. Wash the skin with mild soap and rinse with warm water.
    4. Apply a skin barrier to protect the peristomal skin.
    5. Dry the skin carefully.
    6. Don a pair of clean gloves.

    _____, _____, _____, _____, _____, _____

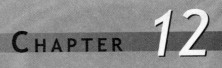

Endocrine Problems

1. A patient is admitted to the medical unit with possible Graves' disease (hyperthyroidism). Which assessment finding supports this diagnosis?
   1. Periorbital edema
   2. Bradycardia
   3. Exophthalmos
   4. Hoarse voice

2. Which change in vital signs would you instruct a nursing assistant to report immediately for a patient with hyperthyroidism?
   1. Increased and rapid heart rate
   2. Decreased systolic blood pressure
   3. Increased respiratory rate
   4. Decreased oral temperature

3. For the patient with hyperthyroidism, what intervention should you delegate to the experienced certified nursing assistant?
   1. Instruct the patient to report palpitations, dyspnea, vertigo, or chest pain.
   2. Check the apical pulse, blood pressure, and temperature every 4 hours.
   3. Draw blood for thyroid-stimulating hormone, T3, and T4 levels.
   4. Explain the side effects of propylthiouracil (PTU) to the patient.

4. As the shift begins, you are assigned these patients. Which patient should you assess first?
   1. A 38-year-old patient with Graves' disease and a heart rate of 94/minute
   2. A 63-year-old patient with type 2 diabetes and fingerstick glucose of 137 mg/dL
   3. A 58-year-old patient with hypothyroidism and heart rate of 48/minute
   4. A 49-year-old patient with Cushing's disease and +1 dependent edema

5. A patient is hospitalized with adrenocortical insufficiency. Which nursing activity should you delegate to the nursing assistant?
   1. Remind patient to change positions slowly.
   2. Check the patient for muscle weakness.
   3. Teach the patient how to collect 24-hour urine.
   4. Plan nursing interventions to promote fluid balance.

6. You assess a patient with Cushing's disease. For which finding will you notify the physician immediately?
   1. Purple striae present on abdomen and thighs
   2. Weight gain of 1 pound since the previous day
   3. +1 dependent edema in ankles and calves
   4. Crackles bilaterally in lower lobes of lungs

7. The patient with pheochromocytoma had surgery to remove his adrenal glands. Which nursing intervention should you delegate to the nursing assistant?
   1. Add strategies to provide a calm and restful environment post-operatively to the care plan.
   2. Warn the patient to avoid smoking and drinking caffeinated beverages.
   3. Monitor the patient's skin and mucous membranes for signs of adequate hydration.
   4. Monitor lying and standing blood pressure every 4 hours with cuff placed on same arm.

8. For the patient with pheochromocytoma, what physical assessment technique should you instruct the LPN/LVN to avoid?

---

9. The patient with adrenal insufficiency is to be discharged taking prednisone 10 mg orally each day. What will you be sure to teach the patient?
   1. Report excessive weigh gain or swelling to the physician.
   2. Rapid changes of position may cause hypotension.
   3. A diet with foods high in potassium may be beneficial.
   4. Signs of hypoglycemia may occur while taking this drug.

10. You are caring for a patient who is post-hypophysectomy for hyperpituitarism. Which post-operative finding requires immediate intervention?
    1. Presence of glucose in nasal drainage
    2. Nasal packing present in nares
    3. Urine output of 40–50 mL per hour
    4. Patient complaints of thirst

11. Which patient's nursing care would be most appropriate for the charge nurse to assign to the LPN, under the supervision of the RN team leader?
    1. A 51-year-old patient with bilateral adrenalectomy just returned from the post-anesthesia care unit
    2. An 83-year-old patient with type 2 diabetes and chronic obstructive pulmonary disease
    3. A 38-year-old patient with myocardial infarction who is preparing for discharge
    4. A 72-year-old patient admitted from long-term care with mental status changes

12. You are providing care for a patient who underwent thyroidectomy 2 days ago. Which laboratory value requires close monitoring?
    1. Calcium
    2. Sodium
    3. Potassium
    4. White blood cells

13. You are preparing to review a teaching plan for a patient with type 2 diabetes. What will you check to determine the patient's level of compliance with his diabetic regimen?
    1. Patient's fasting glucose level
    2. Patient's oral glucose tolerance test results
    3. Patient's glycosylated hemoglobin assay
    4. Patient's fingerstick glucose check for 24 hours

14. The patient has newly diagnosed type 2 diabetes. Which task should you delegate to the nursing assistant?
    1. Arrange consult with the dietitian for patient.
    2. Verify patient's insulin injection technique.
    3. Teach patient to use glucometer for monitoring glucose at home.
    4. Remind patient to check glucose level prior to each meal.

15. A nursing diagnosis for the newly diagnosed diabetic patient is Risk for Injury related to sensory alterations. Which key points should you include in the teaching plan for this patient? (Choose all that apply.)
    1. Clean and inspect your feet every day.
    2. Be sure that your shoes fit properly.
    3. Nylon socks are best to prevent friction between toes and shoes.
    4. Only a podiatrist should trim your toenails.
    5. Report any non-healing skin breaks to your doctor.

16. The diabetic patient has all of these assessment findings. Which will you instruct the LPN/LVN to report immediately?
    1. Fingerstick glucose of 185 mg/dL
    2. Numbness and tingling in both feet
    3. Profuse perspiration
    4. Bunion on left great toe

17. The plan of care for the diabetic patient includes all of the following interventions. Which intervention could you delegate to the nursing assistant?
    1. Check to make sure that the patient's bath water is not too hot.
    2. Discuss community resources for diabetic outpatient care.
    3. Instruct the patient to perform daily foot inspections.
    4. Check the patient's technique for drawing insulin into a syringe.

18. You are precepting a nurse who has recently graduated and passed the NCLEX examination. The new nurse has been on the unit for only 2 days. Which patient should you assign to the new nurse?
    1. A 68-year-old diabetic who is experiencing signs of hyperglycemia including rapid, deep breathing and mental status changes
    2. A 58-year-old diabetic with peripheral neuropathy and cellulitis of the left ankle
    3. A 49-year-old diabetic who has just returned from post-anesthesia care unit (PACU) after a below-the-knee amputation (BKA)
    4. A 72-year-old diabetic with diabetic ketoacidosis (DKA) on an IV insulin drip

19. In the emergency department, during initial assessment of a new admission with diabetes, you discover all of the following. Which information should you immediately report to the physician?
    1. Hammertoe of the left second metatarsophalangeal joint
    2. Rapid respiratory rate with deep inspirations
    3. Numbness and tingling bilaterally in feet and hands
    4. Decreased sensitivity and swelling of the abdomen

20. You are caring for a diabetic patient who is developing DKA. Which delegated task is most appropriate?
    1. Ask the unit clerk to page the physician to come to the unit.
    2. Ask the LPN/LVN to administer IV insulin according to the sliding scale.
    3. Ask the nursing assistant to check the patient's level of consciousness.
    4. Ask the nursing assistant to get the patient a cup of orange juice.

21. A diabetic patient presents with hot and dry skin, rapid and deep respirations, and a fruity odor to his breath. As charge nurse, you observe the new graduate RN accomplishing all these patient tasks. Which one requires that you intervene immediately?
    1. The RN checks the patient's fingerstick glucose.
    2. The RN encourages the patient to drink orange juice.
    3. The RN checks the patient's order for sliding scale insulin.
    4. The RN assesses the patient's vital signs every 15 minutes.

22. You are preparing a 24-year-old patient with diabetes insipidus (DI) for discharge from the hospital. Which statement indicates that the patient needs additional teaching?
    1. "I will drink fluids equal to the amount of my urine output."
    2. "I will weigh myself every day using the same scale."
    3. "I will wear my medical alert bracelet at all times."
    4. "I will gradually wean myself off the vasopressin."

CHAPTER 13

Integumentary Problems

1. You are caring for a client who has just had a squamous cell carcinoma removed from the face. Which of these tasks can you delegate to an experienced nursing LPN/LVN?
   1. Teach the client about risk factors for squamous cell carcinoma.
   2. Show the client how to care for the surgical site at home.
   3. Check for swelling, bleeding, or pain associated with the surgery.
   4. Discuss the reasons for avoiding aspirin use for a week after surgery.

2. As charge nurse in a long-term-care (LTC) facility, you are developing a care plan for a client with a stage 3 pressure ulcer located over the sacrum. Which nursing intervention is most appropriate to delegate to an LPN who works as a team leader in the facility?
   1. Choose the type of dressing to be used on the ulcer.
   2. Use the Norton scale to assess for pressure ulcer risk factors.
   3. Assist the client to change position at frequent intervals.
   4. Inspect and document the appearance of the ulcer daily.

3. You have just received change-of-shift report for the burn unit. Which client should you assess first?
   1. A client with deep partial-thickness burns on both legs who is complaining of severe and continuous leg pain
   2. A client who has just arrived from the emergency department with facial burns associated with a house fire
   3. A client who has just been transferred from the post-anesthesia care unit (PACU) after having skin grafts applied to the anterior chest
   4. A client admitted 3 weeks ago with full-thickness leg and buttock burns who has been waiting for 3 hours to receive discharge teaching

4. You are doing a sterile dressing change for a client with infected deep partial-thickness burns of the chest and abdomen. List the steps of the care plan in the order each should be accomplished.
   1. Apply silver sulfadiazine (Silvadene) ointment.
   2. Obtain aerobic and anaerobic wound cultures.
   3. Administer morphine sulfate 10 mg IV.
   4. Debride wound of eschar using gauze sponges.

   ____, ____, ____, ____

5. You are the nurse-manager in the burn unit. Which client is best assigned to an RN who has floated from the oncology unit?
   1. A 23-year-old who has just been admitted with burns over 30% of the body after a warehouse fire
   2. A 36-year-old who requires discharge teaching about nutrition and wound care after having skin grafts
   3. A 45-year-old with infected partial-thickness back and chest burns who has a dressing change scheduled
   4. A 57-year-old with full-thickness burns on both arms who needs assistance in positioning hand splints

6. You perform a skin assessment on a new resident in an LTC facility. Which of the following is of most concern?
   1. Numerous striae are noted across the abdomen and buttocks.
   2. All the toenails are thickened and yellow in color.
   3. Silver-colored scaling is present on the elbows and knees.
   4. An irregular border is seen on a black mole on the scalp.

7. Which of the following assessment data requires the most immediate further assessment or intervention?
   1. Bluish color around the lips and earlobes
   2. Yellow color of the skin and sclera
   3. Bilateral erythema of the face and neck
   4. Dark brown spotting on the chest and back

8. A 22-year-old female client who has been taking isotretinoin (Accutane) to treat severe cystic acne makes all the following statements while being seen for a routine physical examination. Which statement is of most concern?
   1. "My husband and I are thinking of starting a family soon."
   2. "I don't think there has been much improvement in my skin."
   3. "Sometimes I get nauseated after taking the medication."
   4. "I have been having problems driving when it gets dark."

9. A client is scheduled for patch testing to determine allergies to several substances. Which nursing activities associated with this test are best delegated to a medical assistant working in the allergy clinic?
   1. Explain the purpose of the testing to the client.
   2. Examine the patch area for evidence of a reaction.
   3. Schedule the client to return to the clinic in 2 days for follow-up.
   4. Monitor for anaphylactic reactions after administration of the test.

10. All of these clients are being discharged from the hospital. In planning discharge teaching, for which are you most concerned about the need to use sunscreen?
    1. A 32-year-old with a urinary tract infection who is being discharged with a prescription for tetracycline 250 mg every 6 hours
    2. A fair-skinned 55-year-old who has just had neck surgery and who plans to walk in the yard for 15 minutes 2 times each day
    3. A dark-skinned 62-year-old who has had keloids injected with hydrocortisone
    4. A 78-year-old with a pruritic rash due to an allergic reaction to penicillin

11. As a home health nurse, you are developing the care plan for an elderly client who has just been referred to your agency. One of the nursing diagnoses is Impaired Skin Integrity related to poor nutrition, bladder incontinence, and immobility. Which of the following nursing actions is best to delegate to an experienced nursing assistant who works at the agency?
    1. Tell the client and family to apply the skin barrier cream in a smooth, even layer.
    2. Complete a diet assessment and suggest changes in diet to improve the client's nutrition.
    3. Remind the family to help the client to the commode every 2 hours during the day.
    4. Evaluate the client for improvement in documented areas of skin breakdown or damage.

12. You have prepared a care plan for an elderly client living in an LTC facility who has candidiasis in the skin folds of the abdomen and groin. Which intervention is best for you, as the nurse manager, to delegate to an LPN working in the facility?
    1. Apply nystatin (Mycostatin) powder to the area 3 times daily.
    2. Clean skin folds every 8 hours with mild soap and dry thoroughly.
    3. Evaluate the need for further antifungal treatment at least weekly.
    4. Assess for ongoing risk factors for skin breakdown and infection.

13. A client who is receiving chemotherapy is admitted with widespread herpes simplex lesions of the oral mucosa and lips. The admission assessment data includes a marked recent decrease in oral intake, level 9–10 burning oral pain (0–10 pain scale), and statements by the client indicating emotional distress about the appearance of the lesions. Based on this information, which of these nursing diagnoses is of highest priority?
    1. Risk for Infection related to not knowing how to avoid contacting herpes simplex
    2. Acute Pain related to presence of extensive herpes simplex lesions
    3. Imbalanced Nutrition: Less Than Body Requirements related to decreased oral intake
    4. Disturbed Body Image related to the appearance of the oral lesions

14. A client admitted to the ED complains of itching of the trunk and groin. You note the presence of multiple reddened wheals on the chest, back, and groin. Which question is most appropriate to ask next?
    1. Do you have a family history of eczema?
    2. Have you been using sunscreen regularly?
    3. How do you usually manage stress?
    4. Are you taking any new medications?

15. A 62-year-old client has extensive blister injuries to the back and both legs caused by exposure to toxic chemicals at work and is admitted to the ED. Which of these ordered interventions will you perform first?
    1. Infuse lactated Ringer's solution at 250 mL per hour.
    2. Irrigate the back and legs with 4 L of sterile normal saline.
    3. Obtain blood for a complete blood count and electrolytes.
    4. Document the percentage of total body surface area burned.

16. You have just received the change-of-shift report in the burn unit. Which client requires the most immediate assessment or intervention?
    1. A 22-year-old admitted 4 days previously with facial burns due to a house fire who has been crying since recent visitors left
    2. A 34-year-old who returned from skin-graft surgery 3 hours ago and is complaining of level 8 pain (0–10 pain scale)
    3. A 45-year-old with deep partial-thickness leg burns who has a temperature of 102.6°F and a blood pressure of 98/46
    4. A 57-year-old who was admitted with electrical burns 24 hours ago and has a blood potassium level of 5.6 mEq/L

17. You take the health history for a 60-year-old client who has been admitted to same-day surgery for elective facial dermabrasion. Which information is most important to convey to the plastic surgeon?
    1. The client does not routinely use sunscreen.
    2. The client has a family history of melanoma.
    3. The client has not eaten anything for 8 hours.
    4. The client takes 325 mg of aspirin daily.

18. A newly graduated RN is in the third week of orientation to the medical-surgical unit. Which client is best for you, as charge nurse, to assign to the new graduate?
    1. A 34-year-old who was just admitted to the unit with periorbital cellulitis
    2. A 40-year-old who needs discharge instructions after having skin grafts to the right thigh
    3. A 67-year-old who has a dressing change scheduled after hydrotherapy for a stage 3 pressure ulcer
    4. A 78-year-old who needs teaching before a punch biopsy of a facial lesion

19. An outpatient seen in the clinic for follow-up after being diagnosed with contact dermatitis caused by poison ivy has been taking prednisone (Deltasone) 30 mg daily. You evaluate the client for adverse medication effects. Which information is of most concern?
    1. The client's blood glucose is 136 mg/dL.
    2. The client states, "I am eating all the time."
    3. The client complains of epigastric pain.
    4. The client's blood pressure is 148/84.

20. As charge nurse, you are observing a newly hired RN. Which action by the new RN requires your most immediate action?
    1. Obtaining an anaerobic culture of a superficial partial-thickness arm burn
    2. Administration of tetracycline with a glass of milk to a client with cellulitis
    3. Debridement of a deep partial-thickness burn wound using wet-to-dry dressings
    4. Teaching a newly admitted burn client about the use of pressure garments

CHAPTER 14

Renal and Urinary Problems

1. You are providing nursing care for a 24-year-old female patient admitted to the unit with a diagnosis of cystitis. Which intervention should you delegate to the nursing assistant?
   1. Show the patient how to secure a clean-catch urine sample.
   2. Check the patient's urine for color, odor, and sediment.
   3. Review the nursing care plan and add nursing interventions.
   4. Provide the patient with a clean-catch urine sample container.

2. Which laboratory result is of most concern to you for the adult patient with cystitis?
   1. Serum WBC 9000/mm^3
   2. Urinalysis with 1–2 WBCs present
   3. Urine bacteria 100,000 colonies/mL
   4. Serum hematocrit 36%

3. As charge nurse, which of the following patient's nursing care would you assign to the LPN/LVN, working under the supervision of an RN?
   1. A 48-year-old patient with cystitis who is taking oral antibiotics
   2. A 64-year-old patient with kidney stones and a new order for lithotripsy
   3. A 72-year-old patient with urinary incontinence needing bladder training
   4. A 52-year-old patient with pyelonephritis and severe acute flank pain

4. You are admitting a 66-year-old male patient suspected of having a urinary tract infection. Which piece of the patient's medical history supports this diagnosis?
   1. The patient's wife had a urinary tract infection 1 month ago.
   2. The patient has been followed for prostate disease for 2 years.
   3. The patient had intermittent catheterization 6 months ago.
   4. The patient had a kidney stone removed 1 year ago.

5. The patient's admission diagnosis is rule out interstitial cystitis. Based on anticipated physician's orders, what must your plan of care for this patient include?
   1. Daily urine samples for urinalysis
   2. Accurate intake and output records
   3. Admission urine sample for electrolytes
   4. Teaching about the cystoscopy procedure

6. You are supervising a new graduate RN who is orienting to the unit. The new RN asks why the patient with uncomplicated cystitis is being discharged with orders for ciprofloxacin 250 mg twice a day for only 3 days. What is your best response?
   1. "We should check with the physician as the patient should take this drug for 10 to 14 days."
   2. "A 3-day course of ciprofloxacin is not the appropriate treatment for a patient with uncomplicated cystitis."
   3. "Research has shown that with a 3-day course of ciprofloxacin, there is increased patient adherence to the plan of care."
   4. "Longer courses of antibiotic therapy are required for hospitalized patients to prevent nosocomial infections."

7. Under your supervision, a new graduate RN is teaching the 28-year-old married female patient with cystitis methods to prevent future urinary tract infections. Which statement by the new nurse requires that you intervene?
   1. "You should always drink 1 to 3 liters of fluid every day."
   2. "Empty your bladder regularly even if you do not feel the urge to urinate."
   3. "Drinking cranberry juice daily may decrease bacteria in your bladder."
   4. "It's OK to soak in the tub with bubble bath as it will keep you clean."

8. You are creating a nursing care plan for an elderly patient with incontinence. For which patient will a bladder-training program be an appropriate intervention?
   1. The patient with functional incontinence due to mental status changes
   2. The patient with stress incontinence due to weakened bladder neck support
   3. The patient with urge incontinence and abnormal detrusor muscle contractions
   4. The patient with transient incontinence due to inability to get to toileting facilities

9. The patient with incontinence will be taking oxybutynin chloride (Ditropan) 5 mg by mouth three times a day after discharge. Which information would you be sure to teach this patient prior to discharge?
   1. "Drink fluids or use hard candy when you experience a dry mouth."
   2. "Be sure to notify your physician if you experience a heart rate of less than 60 per minute."
   3. "If necessary, your physician can increase your dose up to 40 mg per day."
   4. "You should take this medication with meals to avoid stomach ulcers."

10. You are providing care for a patient with reflex urinary incontinence. Which action is appropriately delegated to the new LPN/LVN?
    1. Teach the patient bladder emptying by the Credé method.
    2. Demonstrate how to perform intermittent self-catheterization.
    3. Discuss the side effects of bethanechol chloride (Urecholine).
    4. Reinforce the importance of proper handwashing to prevent infection.

11. The patient has urolithiasis and is passing the stones into the lower urinary tract. What is the priority nursing diagnosis for the patient at this time?
    1. Acute Pain
    2. Risk for Infection
    3. Risk for Injury
    4. Fear of Recurrent Stones

12. You are supervising an orienting nurse who is discharging a patient admitted with kidney stones post lithotripsy. Which statement by the nurse requires that you intervene?
    1. "You should finish all of your antibiotics to make sure that you don't get a urinary tract infection."
    2. "Remember to drink at least 3 liters of fluids every day to prevent another stone from forming."
    3. "Report any signs of bruising to your physician immediately as this indicates bleeding."
    4. "You can return to work in 2 days to 6 weeks, depending on what your physician prescribes."

13. As charge nurse, you must rearrange room assignments to admit a new patient. Which two patients are best suited to be roommates?
    1. A 58-year-old patient with urothelial cancer on multiagent chemotherapy
    2. A 63-year-old patient with kidney stones who underwent open ureterolithotomy
    3. A 24-year-old patient with acute pyelonephritis and severe flank pain
    4. A 76-year-old patient with urge incontinence and a urinary tract infection

    3 , 4

14. The patient with polycystic kidney disease (PKD) has the nursing diagnosis Constipation related to compression of intestinal tract. Which nursing care action should you delegate to the newly-trained LPN/LVN?
    1. Explain how to choose foods that are high in fiber.
    2. Explain how to choose foods that promote bowel regularity.
    3. Explore patient's previous bowel problems and bowel routine.
    4. Administer docusate 100 mg by mouth twice a day.

15. You are preparing to insert an intermittent catheter into a male patient to assess for post-void residual urine. Place the following steps in correct order.
    1. Assist patient to the bathroom and ask him to attempt to void.
    2. Retract the foreskin and hold the penis at 60- to 90-degree angle.
    3. Open the catheterization kit and put on sterile gloves.
    4. Lubricate the catheter and insert it through the meatus of the penis.
    5. Position the patient supine in bed or with head slightly elevated.
    6. Drain all urine present in the bladder into the container.
    7. Cleanse the glans penis starting at the meatus and working outward.
    8. Remove the catheter, clean the penis, and measure the amount of urine returned.

    ____, ____, ____, ____, ____, ____, ____, ____

16. You are the admission nurse for a patient with nephrotic syndrome. Which assessment finding supports this diagnosis?
    1. Edema formation
    2. Hypotension
    3. Increased urine output
    4. Flank pain

17. The patient has been diagnosed with renal cell carcinoma (adenocarcinoma of the kidney). You are orienting a new nurse to the unit, who asks why this patient is not receiving chemotherapy. What is your best response?
    1. "The prognosis for this form of cancer is very poor and we will be providing only comfort measures."
    2. "Chemotherapy has been shown to have only limited effectiveness against this type of cancer."
    3. "Research has shown that the most effective means of treating this form of cancer is with radiation therapy."
    4. "Radiofrequency ablation is a minimally invasive procedure that is the best way to treat renal cell carcinoma."

18. You are teaching a patient how best to prevent renal trauma to the right kidney after an injury that required a left nephrectomy. Which of the following points will you include in your teaching plan? (Choose all that apply.)
    1. Always wear a seat belt.
    2. Avoid all contact sports.
    3. Practice safe walking habits.
    4. Wear protective clothing to participate in contact sports.
    5. Use caution when riding a bicycle.

19. You are providing nursing care for a patient with acute renal failure (ARF) who has a nursing diagnosis of Fluid Volume Excess related to compromised regulatory mechanisms. Which actions should you delegate to the experienced nursing assistant? (Choose all that apply.)
    1. Monitor and record vital signs every 4 hours.
    2. Weigh patient every morning using standing scale.
    3. Administer furosemide (Lasix) 40 mg orally twice a day.
    4. Remind patient to save all urine for intake and output record.
    5. Listen to breath sounds every 4 hours.
    6. Ensure that patient's urinal is within reach.

20. The nursing assistant reports to you that the patient with ARF has had a urine output of 350 mL for the past 24 hours after receiving furosemide 40 mg IV push. The nursing assistant asks you how this can happen. What is your best response?
    1. "During the oliguric phase of acute renal failure, patients often do not respond well to either fluid challenges or diuretics."
    2. "There must be some sort of error. Someone must have failed to record the urine output."
    3. "The patient with acute renal failure retains sodium and water, counteracting the action of the furosemide."
    4. "The gradual accumulation of nitrogenous waste products results in the retention of water and sodium."

21. As charge nurse, which patient will you assign to the nurse pulled to your unit from the surgical intensive care unit (SICU)?
    1. Patient with kidney stones scheduled for lithotripsy this morning
    2. Newly post-operative patient with renal stent placement
    3. Newly admitted patient with acute urinary tract infection
    4. Patient with chronic renal failure needing teaching on peritoneal dialysis

22. Your patient is receiving IV piggyback doses of gentamicin every 12 hours. What measurement is your priority for monitoring during the period that the patient is receiving this drug?
    1. Serum creatinine and BUN
    2. Morning weight every day
    3. Intake and output every shift
    4. Temperature elevation

23. The patient with a diagnosis of ARF had a urine output of 1560 mL for the past 8 hours. The LPN/LVN who is caring for this patient under your supervision asks how a patient with renal failure can have such a large urine output. What is your best response?
    1. "The patient's renal failure was due to hypovolemia and we have administered IV fluids to correct the problem."
    2. "Acute renal failure patients go through a diuretic phase when their kidneys begin to recover and may put out up to 10 L of urine per day."
    3. "With that much urine output, there must have been a mistake made when the patient was diagnosed."
    4. "An increase in urine output like this is an indicator that the patient is entering the recovery phase of acute renal failure."

24. The patient on the medical-surgical unit with ARF is to begin continuous veno-venous hemofiltration (CVVH) as soon as possible. What is the priority action at this time?
    1. Call the charge nurse and transfer the patient to the intensive care unit.
    2. Develop a teaching plan for the patient that focuses on CVVH.
    3. Assist the patient with morning bath and mouth care prior to transfer.
    4. Notify the physician that the patient's mean arterial pressure is 68 mm Hg.

CHAPTER 15

Reproductive Problems

1. While working in a long-term-care (LTC) facility, you are assessing a client with a history of benign prostatic hypertrophy (BPH). Which information will require the most immediate action?
   1. Client tells you that he always has trouble starting his urinary stream.
   2. Client's chart shows an elevated prostate-specific antigen (PSA) level.
   3. Client is restless and his bladder is palpable above the symphysis pubis.
   4. Client says he has not voided since having a glass of juice 4 hours ago.

2. While performing a breast examination on a 22-year-old client, you obtain all of these data. Which information is of most concern?
   1. Both breasts have many nodules in the upper, outer quadrants.
   2. Client complains of bilateral breast tenderness with palpation.
   3. The breast on the right side is slightly larger than the left breast.
   4. An irregularly shaped, nontender lump is palpable in the left breast.

3. After having a modified radical mastectomy, a client is transferred to the post-anesthesia care unit (PACU). All of these actions are included in the routine post-operative care for clients who have had this procedure. Which is best to delegate to an experienced LPN?
   1. Monitor client's dressing for any signs of bleeding.
   2. Document the initial assessment on client's chart.
   3. Call client's status report to the charge nurse on the surgical unit.
   4. Teach client about the importance of using pain medication as needed.

4. While working on the hospital surgical unit, you are assigned to care for a client who has had a right breast lumpectomy and axillary lymph node dissection. Which task included in this client's care can you delegate to a nursing assistant?
   1. Teach the client why blood pressure measurements are taken on the left arm.
   2. Elevate the client's arm on two pillows to promote lymphatic drainage.
   3. Assess the client's right arm for lymphedema.
   4. Wrap the client's right arm with elastic bandages.

5. You obtain all of these assessment data about your client with continuous bladder irrigation (CBI) after a transurethral resection of the prostate (TURP). Which information indicates the most immediate need for nursing intervention?
   1. The client states he feels a continuous urge to void.
   2. The catheter drainage is light pink with occasional clots.
   3. The catheter is pulled taut and taped to the client's thigh.
   4. The client complains of painful bladder spasms.

6. A 67-year-old client with incomplete bladder emptying caused by BPH has a new prescription for tamsulosin (Flomax). Which statement about tamsulosin is most important to include when teaching this client?
   1. "This medication will improve your symptoms by shrinking the prostate."
   2. "The force of your urinary stream will probably increase."
   3. "Your blood pressure will decrease as a result of taking this medication."
   4. "You should avoid making sudden changes in position."

7. While working on the surgical unit, you are assigned to care for a client who has just returned to the surgical unit after a TURP. You assess the client and obtain these data. Which finding will require the most immediate action?
   1. Client's blood pressure reading is 153/88.
   2. Client's catheter is draining bright red blood.
   3. Client is not wearing anti-embolism hose.
   4. Client is complaining of abdominal cramping.

8. After a radical prostatectomy, a client is to be discharged with a retention catheter. He has prescriptions for hydrocodone/acetaminophen 5 mg/500 mg (Vicodin) and sulfamethoxazole-trimethoprim (Septra). Which nursing action included in the client discharge plan is best to delegate to an experienced LPN working with you?
   1. Reinforce the need to check his temperature daily.
   2. Demonstrate how to clean around his urinary meatus.
   3. Document a discharge assessment in the client's chart.
   4. Instruct the client about the need to use stool softeners.

9. The day after having a radical prostatectomy, your client has many blood clots in the urinary catheter and states he has frequent bladder spasms. You notice occasional urine leakage around the catheter at the urinary meatus. The client says that his right calf is sore and complains that he feels short of breath. Which action will you take first?
   1. Irrigate the catheter with 50 mL of sterile saline.
   2. Administer oxybutynin (Ditropan) 5 mg orally.
   3. Dorsiflex the foot to check for Homans' sign.
   4. Obtain an oxygen saturation using pulse oximetry.

10. After arriving for your shift in the emergency department (ED), you receive change-of-shift report about all of these clients. Which one do you need to assess first?
    1. A 19-year-old client with scrotal swelling and severe pain that has not decreased with elevation of the scrotum
    2. A 25-year-old client who has a painless indurated lesion on the glans penis
    3. A 44-year-old client with an elevated temperature, chills, and back pain associated with recurrent prostatitis
    4. A 77-year-old client with abdominal pain and acute bladder distention

11. A 79-year-old client who has just returned to the surgical unit following a TURP complains of acute abdominal pain caused by bladder spasms. All of these orders are listed on the client's chart. In what order will you accomplish these actions?
    1. Administer acetaminophen/oxycodone 325 mg/5 mg (Percocet) 2 tablets.
    2. Irrigate retention catheter with 30–50 mL of sterile normal saline.
    3. Infuse 500 mL of 5% dextrose in lactated Ringer's solution over 2 hours.
    4. Encourage client's oral fluid intake to at least 2500–3000 mL daily.

    _____, _____, _____, _____

12. You have obtained these data about a 68-year-old client who is ready for discharge from the ED and has a new prescription for nitroglycerin (Nitro-Stat) 0.4 mg sublingual. Which information about the client has the most immediate implications for client teaching?
    1. The client has benign prostatic hypertrophy and some urinary hesitancy.
    2. The client's father and two brothers all have had myocardial infarctions.
    3. The client uses sildenafil (Viagra) several times weekly for erectile dysfunction.
    4. The client is unable to remember when he first experienced chest pain.

13. You are caring for a 21-year-old client who had a left orchiectomy for testicular cancer on the previous day. Which nursing activities associated with his care will be best to delegate to a new LPN you are orienting to the surgical unit?
    1. Answer the client's questions about the use of chemotherapy and radiation for testicular cancer.
    2. Administer narcotic analgesic medications to the client for pain.
    3. Teach the client how to perform testicular self-examination on the remaining testicle.
    4. Assess the client's knowledge level about the use of sperm banking.

14. You are working as a team with an experienced nursing assistant. Considering your clients' needs for frequent assessments, monitoring, and teaching, which client is most appropriate to assign to the nursing assistant?
    1. A 34-year-old client who has just been admitted with epididymitis and an elevated temperature and needs assessment
    2. A 43-year-old client who needs discharge teaching after having surgery to remove a stage II ovarian cancer
    3. A 50-year-old client who has orders to ambulate in the hallway 2 days after having an abdominal hysterectomy
    4. A 79-year-old client who is receiving continuous bladder irrigation after a transurethral resection of the prostate

15. You have just received change-of-shift report about your assigned clients. In what order will you assess these clients?
    1. A 22-year-old client who has questions about how to care for the drains placed in her breast reconstruction incision
    2. An anxious 44-year-old client who is scheduled to be discharged today after having a total vaginal hysterectomy
    3. A 69-year-old client who is complaining of level 5 pain (0–10 scale) after having a perineal prostatectomy 2 days ago
    4. A usually oriented 78-year-old client who has new-onset confusion after having a bilateral orchiectomy the previous day

    _____, _____, _____, _____

16. After a client has had a needle biopsy of the prostate gland using the transrectal approach, which statement is essential to include in the client teaching plan?
    1. "The doctor will call you about the test results in a day or two."
    2. "Serious infections frequently occur as a complication of this test."
    3. "You will need to call the doctor if you have a fever or chills."
    4. "It is normal to have rectal bleeding for a few days after the test."

17. You are working in the PACU caring for a 32-year-old client who has just arrived after having a dilation and curettage (D&C) to evaluate infertility. Which assessment data are of most concern?
    1. Blood pressure 162/90
    2. Perineal pad saturated after first 30 minutes
    3. O_2 saturation 91%–95%
    4. Sharp, continuous, level 8/10 abdominal pain

18. When developing the plan of care for a home health client who has been discharged after a radical prostatectomy, which activities will you delegate to the home health aide? (Choose all that apply.)
    1. Monitor the client for symptoms of urinary tract infection.
    2. Help the client to connect the catheter to the leg bag.
    3. Assess the client's incision for appropriate wound healing.
    4. Assist the client to ambulate for increasing distances.
    5. Help the client shower at least every other day.

19. You are working in the ED when a client with possible toxic shock syndrome (TSS) is admitted. The physician has given all of these orders. Which one will you implement first?
    1. Remove client's tampon.
    2. Obtain blood cultures from two sites.
    3. Give O_2 at 6 L/minute.
    4. Infuse nafcillin (Unipen) 500 mg IV.

20. When assessing a client with cervical cancer who had a total abdominal hysterectomy yesterday, you obtain the following data. Which information has the most immediate implications for planning the client's care?
    1. Fine crackles are audible at the lung bases.
    2. Client's right calf is swollen and tender.
    3. Client is using the PCA every 15 minutes.
    4. Urine in the collection bag is amber and clear.

21. You observe a student nurse accomplishing all of these activities while caring for a client who has an intracavitary radioactive implant in place to treat cervical cancer. Which action requires that you intervene immediately?
    1. The student stands next to the client for 5 minutes while assisting with her bath.
    2. The student asks the client how she feels about losing her child-bearing ability.
    3. The student assists the client to the bedside commode for a bowel movement.
    4. The student offers to get the client whatever she would like to eat or drink.

22. A 59-year-old woman who had a total abdominal hysterectomy and bilateral salpingo-oophorectomy 3 days ago is complaining of flank pain and a burning sensation with urination. Her total urine output during the previous 8 hours was 210 mL. The client's temperature is 101.3° F. You call the physician to report this information and receive these orders. Which will you implement first?
    1. Insert straight catheter PRN for output less than 300 mL/8 hours.
    2. Administer acetaminophen (Tylenol) 650 mg orally.
    3. Send urine specimen to laboratory for culture and sensitivity.
    4. Administer ceftizoxime (Cefizox) 1 g IV every 12 hours.

23. An 86-year-old woman had an anterior and posterior colporrhaphy (A and P repair) several days ago. The client has been unwilling to ambulate or cough effectively. Her retention catheter was discontinued 8 hours ago. Which information obtained during your assessment has the most immediate implications for her care?
    1. Oral temperature is 100.7° F.
    2. Abdomen is firm and tender to palpation above the symphysis pubis.
    3. Breath sounds are decreased with fine crackles audible at both bases.
    4. Apical pulse is 86 and slightly irregular.

24. While you are orienting a new RN to the medical-surgical unit, you observe the orientee accomplishing all of the following actions while caring for a client with severe pelvic inflammatory disease (PID), who has been admitted to the hospital for administration of IV antibiotics. Which one will require that you intervene most quickly?
    1. The new RN tells the client she should avoid using tampons in the future.
    2. The new RN offers the client an ice pack to decrease her abdominal pain.
    3. The new RN positions the client flat in bed while helping her take a bath.
    4. The new RN teaches the client she should not have intercourse for 2 months.

25. You are administering vancomycin (Vancocin) 500 mg IV to a client with PID when you notice that the client's neck and face are becoming flushed. Which action should you take next?
    1. Discontinue the vancomycin.
    2. Slow the rate of the medication infusion.
    3. Obtain an order for an antihistamine.
    4. Check the client's temperature.

26. Three days after having a pelvic exenteration procedure, a client suddenly complains of a "giving" sensation along her abdominal incision. You check under the dressing and find that the wound edges are open and loops of intestine are protruding. Which action should you take first?
    1. Call the client's surgeon and report that wound evisceration has occurred.
    2. Cover the wound with saline-soaked dressings.
    3. Don sterile gloves and gently replace the intestine back in the wound.
    4. Check the client's blood pressure and heart rate.

27. A client with stage IV ovarian cancer and recurrent ascites is admitted to the medical unit for a paracentesis. Which nursing actions included in the plan of care will you delegate to an LPN who has worked on the medical unit for several years?
    1. Obtain a paracentesis tray from the central supply area.
    2. Complete the short-stay client admission form.
    3. Take vital signs every 15 minutes after the procedure.
    4. Provide discharge instructions after the procedure.

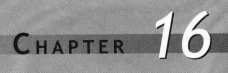

Medical-Surgical Emergencies

1. You are the charge nurse in an emergency department (ED) and must assign two staff members to cover the triage area. Which team is the most appropriate for this assignment?
   1. An advanced practice nurse and an experienced LPN/LVN
   2. An experienced LPN/LVN and an inexperienced RN
   3. An experienced RN and an inexperienced RN
   4. An experienced RN and a nursing assistant

2. You are working in the triage area of an ED, and four patients approach the triage desk at the same time. List the order in which you will assess these patients.
   1. An ambulatory, dazed 25-year-old male with a bandaged head wound
   2. An irritable infant with a fever, petechiae, and nuchal rigidity
   3. A 35-year-old jogger with a twisted ankle, having pedal pulse and no deformity
   4. A 50-year-old female with moderate abdominal pain and occasional vomiting

   ___, ___, ___, ___

3. In conducting a primary survey on a trauma patient, which of the following is considered one of the priority elements of the primary survey?
   1. Complete set of vital signs
   2. Palpation and auscultation of the abdomen
   3. Brief neurologic assessment
   4. Initiation of pulse oximetry

4. A 56-year-old patient presents in triage with left-sided chest pain, diaphoresis, and dizziness. This patient should be prioritized into which category?
   1. High urgent
   2. Urgent
   3. Non-urgent
   4. Emergent

5. The physician has ordered cooling measures for a child with fever who is likely to be discharged when the temperature comes down. Which of the following would be appropriate to delegate to the nursing assistant?
   1. Assist the child to remove outer clothing.
   2. Advise the parent to use acetaminophen instead of aspirin.
   3. Explain the need for cool fluids.
   4. Prepare and administer a tepid bath.

6. It is the summer season, and patients with signs and symptoms of heat-related illness present in the ED. Which patient needs attention first?
   1. An elderly person complains of dizziness and syncope after standing in the sun for several hours to view a parade
   2. A marathon runner complains of severe leg cramps and nausea. Tachycardia, diaphoresis, pallor, and weakness are observed.
   3. A previously healthy homemaker reports broken air conditioner for days. Tachypnea, hypotension, fatigue, and profuse diaphoresis are observed.
   4. A homeless person, poor historian, presents with altered mental status, poor muscle coordination, and hot, dry, ashen skin. Duration of exposure is unknown.

7. You respond to a call for help from the ED waiting room. There is an elderly patient lying on the floor. List the order for the actions that you must perform.
   1. Perform the chin lift or jaw thrust maneuver.
   2. Establish unresponsiveness.
   3. Initiate cardiopulmonary resuscitation (CPR).
   4. Call for help and activate the code team.
   5. Instruct a nursing assistant to get the crash cart.

   ____, ____, ____, ____, ____

8. The emergency medical service (EMS) has transported a patient with severe chest pain. As the patient is being transferred to the emergency stretcher, you note unresponsiveness, cessation of breathing, and no palpable pulse. Which task is appropriate to delegate to the nursing assistant?
   1. Chest compressions
   2. Bag-valve mask ventilation
   3. Assisting with oral intubation
   4. Placing the defibrillator pads

9. An anxious 24-year-old college student complains of tingling sensations, palpitations, and chest tightness. Deep, rapid breathing and carpal spasms are noted. What priority nursing action should you take?
   1. Notify the physician immediately.
   2. Administer supplemental oxygen.
   3. Have the student breathe into a paper bag.
   4. Obtain an order for an anxiolytic medication.

10. An experienced traveling nurse has been assigned to work in the ED; however, this is the nurse's first week on the job. Which area of the ED is the most appropriate assignment for this nurse?
    1. Trauma team
    2. Triage
    3. Ambulatory or fast track clinic
    4. Pediatric medicine team

11. A tearful parent brings a child to the ED for taking an unknown amount of children's chewable vitamins at an unknown time. The child is currently alert and asymptomatic. What information should be immediately reported to the physician?
    1. The ingested children's chewable vitamins contain iron.
    2. The child has been treated several times for ingestion of toxic substances.
    3. The child has been treated several times for accidental injuries.
    4. The child was nauseated and vomited once at home.

12. In caring for a victim of sexual assault, which task is most appropriate for an LPN/LVN?
    1. Assess immediate emotional state and physical injuries.
    2. Collect hair samples, saliva swabs, and scrapings beneath fingernails.
    3. Provide emotional support and supportive communication.
    4. Ensure that the "chain of custody" is maintained.

13. You are caring for a victim of frostbite to the feet. Place the following interventions in the correct order.
    1. Apply a loose, sterile, bulky dressing.
    2. Give pain medication.
    3. Remove the victim from the cold environment.
    4. Immerse the feet in warm water 100°F to 105°F (40.6°C to 46.1°C).

    ___, ___, ___, ___

14. A patient sustains an amputation of the first and second digits in a chainsaw accident. Which task should be delegated to the LPN/LVN?
    1. Gently cleanse the amputated digits with Betadine solution.
    2. Place the amputated digits directly into ice slurry.
    3. Wrap the amputated digits in sterile gauze moistened with saline.
    4. Store the amputated digits in a solution of sterile normal saline.

15. A 36-year-old patient with a history of seizures and medication compliance of phenytoin (Dilantin) and carbamazepine (Tegretol) is brought to the ED by the EMS personnel for repetitive seizure activity that started 45 minutes prior to arrival. You anticipate that the physician will order which drug for status epilepticus?
    1. PO phenytoin and carbamazepine
    2. IV lorazepam (Ativan)
    3. IV carbamazepine
    4. IV magnesium sulfate

16. You are preparing a child for IV conscious sedation prior to repair of a facial laceration. What information should you immediately report to the physician?
    1. The parent is unsure about the child's tetanus immunization status.
    2. The child is upset and pulls out the IV.
    3. The parent declines the IV conscious sedation.
    4. The parent wants information about the IV conscious sedation.

17. An intoxicated patient presents with slurred speech, mild confusion, and uncooperative behavior. The patient is a poor historian but admits to "drinking a few on the weekend." What is the priority nursing action for this patient?
    1. Obtain an order for a blood alcohol level.
    2. Contact the family to obtain additional history and baseline information.
    3. Administer naloxone (Narcan) 2–4 mg as ordered.
    4. Administer IV fluid support with supplemental thiamine as ordered.

18. When an unexpected death occurs in the ED, which of the following tasks is most appropriate to delegate to the nursing assistant?
    1. Escort the family to a place of privacy.
    2. Go with the organ donor specialist to talk to the family.
    3. Assist with postmortem care.
    4. Assist the family to collect belongings.

19. Following emergency endotracheal intubation, you must verify tube placement and secure the tube. List in order the steps that are required to perform this function.
    1. Obtain an order for a chest x-ray to document tube placement.
    2. Secure the tube in place.
    3. Auscultate the chest during assisted ventilation.
    4. Confirm that the breath sounds are equal and bilateral.

    ＿＿＿, ＿＿＿, ＿＿＿, ＿＿＿

20. A teenager arrives by private car. He is alert and ambulatory, but his shirt and pants are covered with blood. He and his hysterical friends are yelling and trying to explain that they were goofing around and he got poked in the abdomen with a stick. Which of the following comments should be given first consideration?
    1. "There was a lot of blood and we used three bandages."
    2. "He pulled the stick out, just now, because it was hurting him."
    3. "The stick was really dirty and covered with mud."
    4. "He's a diabetic, so he needs attention right away."

21. A prisoner, with a known history of alcohol abuse, has been in police custody for 48 hours. Initially, anxiety, sweating, and tremors were noted. Now, disorientation, hallucination, and hyper-reactivity are observed. The medical diagnosis is delirium tremens. What is the priority nursing diagnosis?
    1. Risk for Injury related to seizures
    2. Risk for Other-Directed Violence related to hallucinations
    3. Risk for Situational Low Self-esteem related to police custody
    4. Risk for Nutritional Deficit related to chronic alcohol abuse

22. You are assigned to telephone triage. A patient who was just stung by a common honey bee calls for advice, reports pain and localized swelling, but denies any respiratory distress or other systemic signs of anaphylaxis. What is the first action that you should direct the caller to perform?
    1. Call 911.
    2. Remove the stinger by scraping.
    3. Apply a cool compress.
    4. Take an oral antihistamine.

23. In relation to submersion injuries, which task is most appropriate to delegate to an LPN/LVN?
    1. Talk to a community group about water safety issues.
    2. Stabilize the cervical spine for an unconscious drowning victim.
    3. Remove wet clothing and cover the victim with a warm blanket.
    4. Monitor an asymptomatic near-drowning victim.

24. You are assessing a patient who has sustained a cat bite to the left hand. The cat is up-to-date on immunizations. The date of the patient's last tetanus shot is unknown. Which of the following is the priority nursing diagnosis?
    1. Risk for Infection related to organisms specific to cat bites
    2. Impaired Skin Integrity related to puncture wounds
    3. Ineffective Health Maintenance related to immunization status
    4. Risk for Impaired Mobility related to potential tendon damage

25. These patients present to the ED complaining of acute abdominal pain. Prioritize them in order of severity.
    1. A 35-year-old male complaining of severe, intermittent cramps with three episodes of watery diarrhea, 2 hours after eating
    2. An 11-year-old boy with a low-grade fever, left lower quadrant tenderness, nausea, and anorexia for the past 2 days
    3. A 40-year-old female with moderate left upper quadrant pain, vomiting small amounts of yellow bile, and worsening symptoms over the past week
    4. A 56-year-old male with a pulsating abdominal mass and sudden onset of pressure-like pain in the abdomen and flank within the past hour

    ____, ____, ____, ____

26. The nursing manager decides to form a committee to address the issue of violence against ED personnel. Which combination of employees is best suited to fulfill this assignment?
    1. ED physicians and charge nurses
    2. Experienced RNs and experienced paramedics
    3. RNs, LPN/LVNs, and nursing assistants
    4. At least one representative from each group of ED personnel

27. In a multiple-trauma victim, which assessment finding signals the most serious and life-threatening condition?
    1. A deviated trachea
    2. Gross deformity in a lower extremity
    3. Decreased bowel sounds
    4. Hematuria

28. A patient in a one-car rollover presents with multiple injuries. Prioritize the interventions that must be initiated for this patient.
    1. Secure/start two large-bore IVs with normal saline.
    2. Use the chin lift or jaw thrust method to open the airway.
    3. Assess for spontaneous respirations.
    4. Give supplemental oxygen per mask.
    5. Obtain a full set of vital signs.
    6. Remove patient's clothing.
    7. Insert a Foley catheter if not contraindicated.

    ____, ____, ____, ____, ____, ____, ____

29. In the work setting, what is your primary responsibility in preparing for disaster management that includes natural disasters or bioterrorism incidents?
    1. Knowledge of the agency's emergency response plan
    2. Awareness of the signs and symptoms for potential agents of bioterrorism
    3. Knowledge of how and what to report to the CDC
    4. Ethical decision-making about exposing self to potentially lethal substances

30. You are giving discharge instructions to a woman who has been treated for contusions and bruises sustained during an episode of domestic violence. What is your priority intervention for this patient?
    1. Transportation arrangements to a safe house
    2. Referral to a counselor
    3. Advise about contacting the police
    4. Follow-up appointment for injuries

31. Emergency and ambulatory care nurses are among the first health care workers to encounter victims from a bioterrorist attack. Prioritize the actions for the ED staff in the event of a biochemical incident.
    1. Report to the public health department or CDC per protocol.
    2. Decontaminate the victims in a separate area.
    3. Protect the environment for the safety of personnel and non-affected patients.
    4. Don personal protective equipment.
    5. Triage according to protocol.

    ____, ____, ____, ____, ____

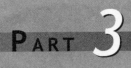
Prioritization, Delegation, and Assignment in Complex Health Scenarios

Chest Pressure, Indigestion, Nausea, and Vomiting

Ms. S. is a 58-year-old African-American woman who was admitted to the coronary care unit (CCU) from the emergency department (ED) with complaints of chest pressure and indigestion associated with nausea and vomiting. She started feeling ill about 3 hours prior to admission. She tells the nurse that she tried drinking water and took some Pepto-Bismol that she had in her bathroom medicine cabinet. She has also tried lying down to rest, but none of these actions helped. She states, "It just gets worse and worse." Ms. S. has been under a physician's care for the past 12 years for management of hypertension and swelling in her ankles. She was a smoker, but quit 1 year ago.

In the ED, admission laboratory tests, including cardiac enzymes, were drawn and a 12-lead electrocardiogram (ECG) was done.

CCU admission vital signs are:

Blood pressure	174/92
Heart rate	120–130 beats per minute, irregular
Temperature	99.8°F oral
Respirations	30–34 breaths per minute
Pulse oximetry	Sao_2 94% on room air

1. You may delegate which action to a nursing assistant?
   1. Place the client on a cardiac telemetry monitor.
   2. Draw cardiac enzymes and send to laboratory.
   3. Obtain a 12-lead electrocardiogram.
   4. Monitor and record client's intake and output.

2. Which of the physician's orders takes first priority at this time?
   1. Check vital signs every 2 hours.
   2. Obtain 12-lead ECG every 6 hours.
   3. Place client on cardiac monitor.
   4. Check cardiac enzymes every 6 hours.

3. What is the cardiac isoenzyme that rises early and is most specific in detecting early acute heart attack?

4. The client's telemetry cardiac monitor shows a rhythm of sinus tachycardia with frequent premature ventricular contractions (PVCs). Which drug should you administer first?
   1. amiodarone (Cordarone) IV push
   2. nitroglycerin sublingually
   3. morphine sulfate IV push
   4. atenolol (Tenormin) IV push

5. All of the following laboratory values were obtained in the ED. Which value has immediate implications for the care of this client?
   1. Potassium 3.4
   2. CK 329/CK-MB 7%
   3. Glucose 123
   4. Slight elevation of WBCs

6. Ms. S. complains of worsening chest discomfort. The cardiac monitor shows ST segment elevation and you notify the physician. Which of the following orders takes priority?
   1. Administer morphine sulfate 2 mg IV push.
   2. Schedule an echocardiogram.
   3. Draw serum coagulation studies.
   4. Give ranitidine 75 mg orally every 12 hours.

7. Because Ms. S. continues to experience chest pain and has elevated cardiac enzymes, the following interventions have been ordered. What interventions can you assign to an experienced nursing assistant? (Choose all that apply.)
   1. Take vital signs every 2 hours.
   2. Maintain accurate intake and output.
   3. Administer tenecteplase IV push.
   4. Conduct serum coagulation studies.
   5. Read cardiac monitor every 4 hours.
   6. Assist her to the bedside commode.

8. You delegate to the nursing assistant the task of taking the client's vital signs every 2 hours and recording the vital signs in the electronic chart. Later you check the client's chart and discover that the vital signs have not been recorded. What is your best action?
   1. Take the vital signs because it is not within the nursing assistant's scope of practice.
   2. Notify the nurse manager immediately.
   3. Call the nursing assistant to the nurses' station to reprimand.
   4. Speak to the nursing assistant privately to determine why the vital signs were not recorded.

9. Ms. S. is stable and has been transferred to the cardiac step-down unit. Which of the following should you instruct the nursing assistant to report immediately?
   1. Temperature elevation to 99°F, with morning vital signs
   2. Chest pain episode occurring during morning care
   3. Blood pressure increase of 10 mm Hg after morning care
   4. Heart rate increase, 10 beats per minute after ambulation

10. The physician orders captopril (Capoten) 12.5 mg PO twice daily and hydrochlorothiazide (HCTZ) 25 mg PO every day. Which of the following would you be sure to include when teaching the client about these drugs?
    1. "Take your hydrochlorothiazide in the morning."
    2. "If you miss a dose of captopril, take two tablets next time."
    3. "Avoid foods that are rich in potassium."
    4. "You should expect an increase in blood pressure."

Dyspnea and Shortness of Breath

Mr. W. is an 83-year-old man who was brought into the hospital from a long-term care facility by the paramedics, complaining of severe dyspnea and shortness of breath. He has been experiencing cold-like symptoms for the past 2 days. He has a productive cough with thick greenish sputum. Mr. W. woke up in the nursing home and found that he was having difficulty breathing even after using his albuterol metered dose inhaler (MDI). He appears very anxious and is in respiratory distress. His history includes chronic obstructive pulmonary disease (COPD) related to smoking two packs of cigarettes per day since he was 15 years old. Mr. W. has been incontinent of urine and stool for the past 2 years.

In the emergency department, the patient had a chest x-ray, as well as admission laboratory tests, including electrolytes and a complete blood count (CBC). A sputum sample was sent to the laboratory for culture, sensitivity, and Gram stain.

Vital Signs:	Temperature:	100.9°F orally
	Respirations:	38/minute
	Heart rate:	118/minute
	Blood pressure:	154/92
	Pulse oximetry:	Sao_2 88% on 1 L/minute oxygen by nasal cannula

1. What is the priority nursing diagnosis for this patient?
   1. Decreased Cardiac Output
   2. Ineffective Breathing Pattern
   3. Anxiety
   4. Acid-base Imbalance

2. Below are the physician's orders for this patient. Which intervention should the nurse complete first?
   1. Send arterial blood gas sample to the laboratory.
   2. Schedule pulmonary function tests.
   3. Repeat chest x-ray each morning.
   4. Give albuterol MDI 2 puffs every 4 hours.

The patient's arterial blood gas results include pH: 7.37, PaCO_2: 55.4, PaO_2: 51.2, HCO_3^-: 38, O_2 saturation: 82%. These results are interpreted as compensated respiratory acidosis with hypoxemia.

3. Which of the following interventions would you assign to an experienced LPN?
   1. Draw arterial blood gas sample.
   2. Administer albuterol by hand-held nebulizer.
   3. Take vital signs every 2 hours.
   4. Increase oxygen to 2 L per nasal cannula.

4. Which interventions could you delegate to a new nursing assistant? (Choose all that apply.)
   1. Assist the patient in using a bedside commode.
   2. Check pulse oximetry every shift.
   3. Teach the patient to cough and deep breathe.
   4. Remind the patient to use incentive spirometry every 4 hours.
   5. Assess the patient's breath sounds every shift.
   6. Encourage the patient to drink adequate oral fluids.

5. During morning rounds, the nurse notes all of the following assessment findings. Which finding indicates worsening of the patient's condition?
   1. Barrel-shaped chest
   2. Clubbed fingers on both hands
   3. Crackles bilaterally
   4. Frequent productive cough

6. You report your morning assessment findings (see Question #5) to the physician. Which physician's order is most directly related to your findings?
   1. Administer furosemide (Lasix) 20 mg IV push now.
   2. Record accurate intake and output.
   3. Administer potassium 20 mEq orally every morning.
   4. Weigh the patient every morning.

7. Which assessment would you instruct the nursing assistant to report immediately?
   1. Patient was incontinent of urine and stool.
   2. Patient has lost 1 pound since admission.
   3. Patient has increased elevation of temperature.
   4. Patient ate only half of breakfast and lunch.

8. The nursing assistant took morning vital signs on this patient and immediately reported the following to you. Which takes priority when notifying the physician?
   1. Heart rate 96 per minute
   2. Blood pressure 160/90
   3. Respiratory rate 34 per minute
   4. Temperature 103.5°F orally

9. The LPN tells you that the patient is now on oxygen at 2 L/minute by nasal cannula and his pulse oximetry reads 91%. What intervention should you delegate to the LPN?
   1. Begin a plan for discharging the patient.
   2. Administer furosemide 20 mg orally each morning.
   3. Get a baseline weight on the patient now.
   4. Administer IV piggy-back cefotaxime (Claforan) every 6 hours.

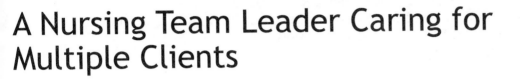

A Nursing Team Leader Caring for Multiple Clients

You are the team leader providing care for six clients. The team includes yourself (an RN), an LPN/LVN, and a newly hired nursing assistant, who is orienting to the unit. The six clients are:

- *Mr. C., a 68-year-old man with unstable angina who needs teaching for a cardiac catheterization scheduled this morning*
- *Ms. J., a 45-year-old woman experiencing chest pain scheduled for a graded exercise test later today*
- *Mr. R., a 75-year-old man with 4-day-old left-sided stroke*
- *Ms. S., an 83-year-old woman with heart disease, a history of myocardial infarction, and mild dementia*
- *Ms. B., a 93-year-old woman, newly admitted from long-term care with decreased urine output, altered level of consciousness, and an elevated temperature of 99.5° F*
- *Mr. L., a 59-year-old man with mild shortness of breath and chronic emphysema*

1. Which clients should you assign to the LPN for nursing care tasks under your supervision? (Choose all that apply.)
   1. Mr. C.
   2. Ms. J.
   3. Mr. R.
   4. Ms. S.
   5. Ms. B.
   6. Mr. L.

2. Which client should you assess first?
   1. Mr. C.
   2. Ms. J.
   3. Ms. B.
   4. Mr. L.

3. Which of these is a key point to include when teaching the client about the post-procedure care for a cardiac catheterization?
    1. "There are no restrictions after the procedure."
    2. "We will get you out of bed within 2 hours after the procedure."
    3. "You will have to stay flat in bed for 6 to 8 hours."
    4. "Family visitors will be restricted until the next day."

4. The physician's orders for Ms. J., who is experiencing chest pain, are as follows. List the orders in the sequence that they should be completed. (Answers may be used more than once).
    1. Obtain 12-lead electrocardiogram (ECG) when client experiences chest pain.
    2. Administer nitroglycerin 0.6 mg SL as needed for chest pain every 5 minutes times 3.
    3. Administer morphine 2 mg IV push as needed for chest pain.
    4. Monitor blood pressure and heart rate.

    _4_, _1_, _2_, ____, ____, ____, ____, ____, ____, ____

5. Which of the following should you delegate to the nursing assistant?
    1. Ask Ms. S. memory-testing questions.
    2. Tell Ms. J. about treadmill exercise testing.
    3. Check pulse oximetry for Mr. L.
    4. Monitor urine output for Ms. B.

6. The nursing assistant is delegated the task of taking morning vital signs for all six clients. What would you instruct the nursing assistant to report immediately?
    1. Temperature greater than 102°F orally
    2. Blood pressure greater than 140/80 mm Hg
    3. Heart rate of 60 beats per minute
    4. Respiratory rate less than 18 per minute

7. The nursing assistant asks why it is important to notify someone whenever a client with heart disease complains of chest pain. What is your best response?
    1. "It's important to keep track of the chest pain episodes so we can notify the physician."
    2. "The client may need morphine to alleviate the chest pain."
    3. "Chest pain may indicate coronary artery blockage and heart muscle damage."
    4. "Our unit policy includes specific steps to take in the treatment of clients with chest pain."

8. The physician's orders for Mr. R. (the client with a stroke) include assisting the client with meals. To whom should you delegate this task?
    1. Physical therapist
    2. Nursing assistant
    3. LPN/LVN
    4. Occupational therapist

9. The nursing assistant tells you that Mr. L., the client with chronic emphysema, stated that he is feeling short of breath after walking to the bathroom. What action should you take at this time?
    1. Notify the physician.
    2. Increase oxygen flow to 4 L by nasal cannula.
    3. Assess oxygen saturation by pulse oximetry.
    4. Remind the client to cough and deep breathe.

10. Ms. B.'s oral temperature is now 102.6°F. What is your best action?
    1. Notify the physician.
    2. Administer acetaminophen 2 tablets orally.
    3. Ask the LPN/LVN to give an acetaminophen suppository.
    4. Remove extra blankets from the client's bed.

11. What factor most likely precipitated Ms. B.'s elevated temperature?

    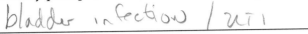 bladder infection / UTI

12. You are working on a nursing care plan for Ms. B., the client newly admitted from long-term care with decreased urine output and altered level of consciousness. Which nursing intervention is most appropriate to delegate to the nursing assistant?
    1. Check client's level of consciousness every shift.
    2. Assist with ambulation to the bathroom to void.
    3. Teach the client the side effects of antibiotic therapy.
    4. Administer a sulfonamide orally every 12 hours.

13. The nursing assistant reports that Mr. L.'s heart rate, which was 86 per minute in the morning, is now 98 per minute. What would be the most appropriate question to ask Mr. L.?
    1. "Have you just returned from the bathroom?"
    2. "Did you recently use your albuterol inhaler?"
    3. "Are you feeling short of breath?"
    4. "How much do you smoke?"

14. The LPN/LVN reports that Ms. S. will not leave the chest leads for her cardiac monitor in place and asks if she can restrain the client. What is your best response?
    1. "Yes, this client had a heart attack and we must keep her on the cardiac monitor."
    2. "Yes, but be sure to use soft restraints so that the client's circulation is not compromised."
    3. "No, we must have a physician's order before we can apply restraints in any situation."
    4. "No, but try covering the lead wires with the sheet so that the client does not see them."

15. Close to the end of the shift, the LPN/LVN reports that the nursing assistant has not totaled clients' intake and output for the past 8 hours. What is your best action?
    1. Confront the nursing assistant and instruct her to complete this assignment.
    2. Delegate this task to the LPN/LVN as the nursing assistant may not have been educated in this task.
    3. Ask the nursing assistant if she needs assistance completing the intake and output records.
    4. Notify the nurse manager to include this on the nursing assistant's evaluation.

16. The 5 Rights guide delegation of nursing care tasks. As team leader, list the 5 Rights.

    _____

    _____

    _____

    _____

    _____

Shortness of Breath, Edema, and Decreased Urine Output

Ms. J. is a 63-year-old woman who is admitted directly to the medical unit after visiting her physician for shortness of breath and increased swelling in her ankles and calves. Her admitting diagnosis is rule out chronic renal failure (CRF). Ms. J. states that her symptoms have become worse over the past two to three months and that she uses the bathroom less often and urinates in smaller amounts. Her past medical history includes hypertension (30 years), coronary artery disease (18 years), and type 2 diabetes (14 years).

Admission vital signs:	Temperature	97.8°F
	Blood pressure	162/96
	Heart rate	88/minute
	Respiratory rate	28/minute
	Pulse oximetry	91% on room air

Admission laboratory tests to be collected on the unit include serum electrolytes, renal function tests, complete blood count (CBC), and urinalysis. A 24-hour urine collection for creatinine clearance has also been ordered.

1. During admission assessment, Ms. J. has all of these findings. For which finding should you notify the physician immediately?
   1. 2+ Bilateral pitting ankle and calf edema
   2. Crackles in both lower and middle lobes
   3. Dry and peeling skin on both feet
   4. Faint but palpable pedal and post-tibial pulses

2. Which task, associated with a 24-hour urine collection, is appropriate to delegate to the nursing assistant?
   1. Instruct Ms. J. to collect all urine with each voiding.
   2. Explain the purpose of collecting urine for 24 hours.
   3. Ensure that the 24-hour urine collection is kept on ice.
   4. Review Ms. J.'s urine for color, odor, and sediment.

3. You review Ms. J.'s laboratory results. Which laboratory result is of most concern?
   1. Serum potassium 7.2 mmol/L
   2. Serum creatinine 15 mg/dL
   3. Blood urea nitrogen 180 mg/dL
   4. Serum calcium 7.8 mg/dL

4. Which medication should you be prepared to administer to lower the patient's potassium?
   1. furosemide 40 mg IV push
   2. erythropoietin 300 U/kg subcutaneously
   3. calcium 1 tablet by mouth
   4. sodium polystyrene sulfonate 15 g by mouth

5. You are the team leader, supervising an LPN/LVN. Which nursing care action for Ms. J. should you delegate to the LPN/LVN?
   1. Insert an intermittent catheter to assess for residual urine.
   2. Plan fluid restriction amounts to be given with meals.
   3. Check breath sounds for presence of increased crackles.
   4. Discuss renal replacement therapies with the patient.

6. As team leader, you observe the nursing assistant (NA) perform all of these actions for Ms. J. For which action must you intervene?
   1. NA assists Ms. J. to replace oxygen nasal cannula.
   2. NA checks Ms. J.'s vital signs after the patient drinks fluids.
   3. NA ambulates with Ms. J. to the bathroom and back.
   4. NA washes Ms. J.'s back, legs, and feet with warm water.

7. Ms. J's nursing care plan includes the nursing diagnosis Fluid Volume Excess. What interventions are appropriate for this nursing diagnosis? (Choose all that apply.)
   1. Measure weight daily.
   2. Review daily intake and output.
   3. Restrict sodium intake with meals.
   4. Restrict fluid to 1500 mL plus urine output.
   5. Assess for crackles and edema every shift.

8. After discussing renal replacement therapies with the physician and nurse, Ms. J. is considering hemodialysis (HD). Which statement indicates that Ms. J. needs additional teaching about HD?
   1. "I will need surgery to create an access for hemodialysis."
   2. "I will be able to eat and drink what I want once I start dialysis."
   3. "I will have a temporary dialysis access for a few months."
   4. "I will be having dialysis three times every week."

9. You are supervising a new orienting nurse providing care for Ms. J., who has had surgery to create a left forearm dialysis access. Which of the actions performed by the nurse requires that you intervene?
   1. The nurse monitors the patient's operative site dressing for evidence of bleeding.
   2. The nurse obtains blood pressure reading by placing the cuff on the right arm.
   3. The nurse draws post-operative laboratory studies from temporary dialysis access.
   4. The nurse administers oxycodone by mouth for moderate post-operative pain.

10. Assessment of Ms. J. after dialysis reveals all of these findings. Which assessment finding necessitates immediate action?
    1. Ms. J.'s weight is decreased by 4.5 pounds.
    2. Ms. J.'s systolic blood pressure is decreased by 14 mm Hg.
    3. Ms. J.'s level of consciousness is decreased.
    4. Ms. J.'s temporary catheter dressing has a small blood spot.

11. Six months later, Ms. J. is readmitted to the unit. She has just returned from HD. Which nursing care action should you delegate to the nursing assistant?
    1. Obtain vital signs and post-dialysis weight.
    2. Assess HD access site for bruit and thrill.
    3. Check access site dressing for bleeding.
    4. Instruct patient to request assistance getting out of bed.

12. Ms. J. is preparing for discharge. You are supervising the student nurse who is teaching the patient about her discharge medications. For which statement by the student nurse will you intervene?
    1. "Your Renagel prevents your body from absorbing phosphorus."
    2. "You should take your folic acid after dialysis on dialysis days."
    3. "The docusate is to prevent constipation that may be caused by ferrous sulfate."
    4. "You must take the Epogen three times a week by mouth to treat anemia."

Abdominal Pain, Polyuria, Vomiting, and Thirst

Mr. D., a 19-year-old college student, was brought to the emergency department (ED) by his roommate. He reports abdominal pain, polyuria for the past 2 days, vomiting several times prior to arrival, and subjective thirst. He appears flushed, and his lips and mucous membranes are dry and cracked. His skin turgor is poor. He demonstrates deep rapid respirations; there is a fruity odor to his breath. He is a type 1 diabetic and "may have skipped a few doses of insulin because of cramming for finals." He is alert and conversant but is having trouble focusing on your questions.

Vital signs:		
	Blood pressure	110/60
	Pulse	110/min
	Respirations	32/min
	Temperature	100.8°F
	Accu-Check	685 mg/dL

1. To clarify pertinent data, what questions are appropriate to ask Mr. D.? (Choose all that apply.)
    1. "When did your symptoms start?"
    2. "How many times have you vomited?"
    3. "What was the reading of your last blood sugar?"
    4. "Why didn't you go to see your doctor sooner?"
    5. "Where does your abdomen hurt?"
    6. "Did you take any insulin today?"
    7. "Do you have any allergies?"

2. You have completed triage assessment and history. What now is your priority action?
    1. Page the ED physician STAT to triage.
    2. Call the client's parents for permission to treat.
    3. Notify the client's primary care physician.
    4. Send the client to the waiting room.
    5. Take the client immediately to a treatment room.

3. What is the priority nursing diagnosis for Mr. D.?
    1. Breathing Pattern, Ineffective related to acidosis
    2. Anxiety related to uncertainty of outcomes
    3. Deficient Fluid Volume related to hyperglycemia
    4. Noncompliance related to medications and treatment plan

4. Which task(s) is (are) appropriate to assign to the experienced nursing assistant? (Choose all that apply.)
   1. Check Mr. D.'s hourly vital signs.
   2. Check Mr. D.'s blood sugar.
   3. Bag and label Mr. D.'s belongings.
   4. Update the roommate on Mr. D.'s status.
   5. Measure and record Mr. D.'s emesis.

5. In caring for Mr. D., what immediate interventions do you anticipate the physician will order? (Choose all that apply.)
   1. Start a peripheral IV with a large-bore catheter.
   2. Insert a Foley catheter with a urinometer.
   3. Give regular insulin subcutaneously.
   4. Have Mr. D. slowly sip isotonic fluids.
   5. Maintain Mr. D. in a semi- or high-Fowler's position.
   6. Give supplemental O_2 per cannula or mask

6. What do you anticipate the physician will order for initial fluid replacement?
   1. Normal saline (0.9% sodium chloride)
   2. D_5W (dextrose 5% in water)
   3. Half-strength saline (0.45% sodium chloride)
   4. Normal saline with KCl (potassium chloride)

7. Within the first 4 hours of initiating therapy for Mr. D., which serum potassium level would concern you the most?
   1. Potassium 3.5 mEq/L
   2. Potassium 2.9 mEq/L
   3. Potassium 5.8 mEq/L

8. The physician has ordered insulin therapy for Mr. D. Place the steps of preparation and administration in the correct order.
   1. Begin the infusion at 0.1 unit/kg/hr.
   2. Prime the correct tubing with normal saline.
   3. Thread the tubing through the IV pump.
   4. Add 100 units of insulin to 100 mL normal saline.
   5. Label the bag with the type and amount of insulin.
   6. Draw up 100 units of regular insulin; other RN checks dose.
   7. Give an IV bolus of regular insulin as ordered.

   ____, ____, ____, ____, ____, ____, ____

9. You are trying to call report to the intensive care unit (ICU) but are told "They have not been notified about the admission." You call the admitting clerk, but she says, "I was never notified." You ask the unit secretary and he tells you, "I forgot to do it." What should you do first?
   1. Report the unit secretary to the manager.
   2. Ask the secretary to call the admissions office now.
   3. Take the secretary aside and allow him to explain his actions.
   4. Ask the ICU to take report regardless of the clerical omission.

10. Which tasks can you delegate to the experienced nursing assistant to facilitate Mr. D.'s transfer to ICU? (Choose all that apply.)
    1. Give the roommate directions to the ICU waiting room.
    2. Independently transport Mr. D. to ICU.
    3. Collect and organize the chart and laboratory reports.
    4. Obtain a portable O$_2$ tank and cardiac monitor.
    5. Place Mr. D. on the portable cardiac monitor.
    6. Obtain the last set of vital signs.

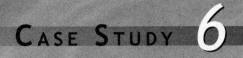

Home Health

You are working as a staff nurse for the home health division of a public health agency. You arrive for the day with plans to make home visits to all six of the following patients:

- ✓ *Ms. A., a patient with chronic obstructive pulmonary disease (COPD) who called the agency saying she has been feeling more dyspneic and has been turning up her home oxygen flow rate*
- *Mr. D., a diabetic patient living alone who is scheduled for a weekly assessment of a chronic leg infection and has daily home health aide visits*
- *Ms. F., an elderly patient whose daughter helps her with peritoneal dialysis and who is due for her three-times-weekly epoetin alfa (Procrit) injection*
- ✓ *Mr. I., a patient who is receiving outpatient chemotherapy and needs a complete blood count (CBC) drawn during his nadir to check his bone marrow function (The nadir is the time when bone marrow and white blood cell counts are at their lowest levels after chemotherapy.)*
- ✓ *Ms. R., a patient with an acute myocardial infarction (MI) who was discharged yesterday from the hospital and needs an initial admission assessment*
- *Mr. S., a patient with multiple sclerosis who was recently hospitalized with pneumonia and is ready for discharge from home health*

1. Soon after you arrive, your manager tells you about a required case management in-service today at 2:00 PM. You realize that you will only have time to make four visits before the in-service. Which four patients will you schedule to see today?

   _____Ms A_____

   _____Ms R._____

   _____Mr I_____

   _____Ms F_____

2. You have adjusted your schedule to visit these four patients today. Which patient will you see first?
   1. Ms. A., the patient with COPD and increased shortness of breath
   2. Ms. F., the peritoneal dialysis patient who will need an epoetin injection
   3. Mr. I., the chemotherapy patient who will need blood drawn for a CBC
   4. Ms. R., the patient with a recent MI who will need an initial assessment

3. You call the four patients to confirm the visits and schedule times. All goes well, until you call Ms. R. to schedule a visit. She says that she doesn't have much time today, but will be available for longer tomorrow. What is the best response?
   1. "The visit will not take very long, so I will plan on seeing you today."
   2. "I have rescheduled other patients because it is essential that I assess you today."
   3. "Perhaps you are feeling that you do not really need any help at home."
   4. "Because of your new heart attack, I would like to visit as soon as possible."

After obtaining Ms. R.'s consent for a visit later today, you head off to see Ms. A. Her husband answers the door and tells you that Ms. A. is resting so comfortably that he does not want you to disturb her. He explains, "She has been so short of breath lately that this is the best sleep she has had in a while."

You talk him into allowing you to assess Ms. A. and find that she is very difficult to awaken. She tries to respond to your questions, but her speech is so slurred you are unable to understand her. The flow meter on her home oxygen is set at 6 L/minute.

4. Which nursing action is most appropriate next?
   1. Auscultate Ms. A.'s anterior and posterior lung sounds.
   2. Check Ms. A.'s oxygen saturation using pulse oximetry.
   3. Continue to stimulate Ms. A. until she can respond to you.
   4. Call the physician and report Ms. A.'s change in status.

5. You obtain an oxygen saturation of 99% with the pulse oximeter. Which action is appropriate now?
   1. Discontinue the oxygen because the high flow is contributing to her somnolence. *Decrease the high flow O₂*
   2. Draw arterial blood gases in order to check her pH, Pao_2, and $Paco_2$ levels.
   3. Call the patient's physician and obtain an order to transport Ms. A to the hospital.
   4. Remind Ms. A.'s husband about the reasons for using oxygen at low flow rates.

When you call the physician to discuss Ms. A.'s status and your actions, you receive an order to have her admitted to the hospital medical unit for further evaluation.

After calling a brief report to the charge nurse on the hospital medical unit, you leave to make the scheduled visit to Ms. R. On the way, you receive a phone call from Mr. D.'s home health aide. Mr. D. is complaining of generalized aches and pains. In addition, his morning blood glucose was 306 mg/dL and he has a temperature of 100.1°F.

6. You realize that Mr. D. will require an assessment today and that you need to reschedule one of your planned patient visits. Which one of the three patients that you were planning to visit today is best to reschedule for tomorrow?

   _____ Ms F _____

7. After rescheduling your patient, you arrive at Ms. R.'s home as arranged and she greets you at the door. You notice that her respiratory effort seems a little labored and she looks anxious. After you introduce yourself to Ms. R., you ask her how she has been feeling since her discharge from the hospital yesterday. Which response indicates a need for immediate intervention?
   1. "I have been a bit short of breath."
   2. "I feel a slight chest pressure."
   3. "I don't understand why I need to take all these pills."
   4. "I am confused about why you are here to see me."

8. Five minutes after taking a nitroglycerin (Nitro-Stat) sublingual tablet, Ms. R. tells you that the chest pressure is "almost gone." Which action should you take next?
   1. Proceed with assessing her and completing the admission documentation.
   2. Have her rest for another 5 minutes and then reassess the chest pressure.
   3. Check her blood pressure and administer another nitroglycerin tablet.
   4. Call the physician, anticipating an order to readmit her to the hospital.

After a second nitroglycerin tablet, Ms. R. says that the chest pressure is completely gone and you proceed to obtain a health history and admission assessment. She lives alone, but her daughter, who lives 20 miles away, visits her about twice a week. Her daughter arrives while you are assessing Ms. R. and stays for the rest of the visit. The house is cluttered and Ms. R.'s hair is uncombed. She says she is too tired to get in and out of the bathtub, so she tries to clean up at the bathroom sink every day.

You find that Ms. R. has crackles at the bases of both lungs and 2+ pedal edema. She has had the chest pressure twice since her discharge yesterday, but, "I just waited and it went away after an hour or so." She has not been taking her prescribed medications, because, "I can't remember which ones I have taken and I don't want to take an overdose." She has many questions about her medications. Her medications include:

- *nitroglycerin (Nitro-Stat) 0.4 mg SL as needed for chest pain*
- *transdermal nitroglycerin (Nitro-Dur) 0.2 mg/hour every morning*
- *metoprolol (Toprol XL) 25 mg PO daily*
- *aspirin (Ecotrin) 81 mg PO daily*
- *enalapril (Vasotec) 2.5 mg PO daily*

9. Based on the information you have obtained, you develop a care plan. Which of the nursing activities will you delegate to a home health aide? (Choose all that apply.)
   1. Set up Ms. R.'s medications in a multi-dose pill box twice a week.
   2. Instruct the daughter how to set up Ms. R.'s daily medications.
   3. Teach Ms. R. and her daughter the purpose for each medication.
   4. Assist Ms. R. with a bath and personal hygiene every day.
   5. Check vital signs daily.
   6. Weigh the patient daily.
   7. Auscultate lung and heart sounds weekly.
   8. Check for any peripheral edema weekly.

10. You assist Ms. R. with taking her scheduled medications for today and remind the patient and her daughter to use the Nitro-Stat tablets if she develops any more chest pressure or pain. The daughter says she will stay with Ms. R. the rest of the day. You instruct the patient and her daughter that Ms. R. should call the doctor or go to the emergency department (ED) if she develops more dyspnea or has chest pain that is unrelieved by three nitroglycerin tablets. Prior to leaving, you make arrangements with Ms. R. for the next visit. When will you schedule the next home visit?
    1. Later today, because Ms. R.'s condition is very unstable and she may require hospital readmission.
    2. Tomorrow, because Ms. R.'s assessment indicates that she needs frequent evaluation and/or interventions.
    3. In 3 days, because the home health aide will see Ms. R. every day and will call you if there are any further problems.
    4. Early the next week, so that there will be enough time to evaluate the effect of the medications on Ms. R's symptoms.

Mr *, chemo*

11. You still have visits to make to Mr. D. and Mr. I. before the mandatory in-service. Which patient will you visit first?

_____Mr I before Mr D_____

You check your cell phone while driving to your next visit and see that your nurse manager has called you. When you call back, the manager tells you about a newly referred 70-year-old patient with emphysema who will need an initial visit today in order to evaluate the need for home oxygen therapy.

12. Since you will not have time today to visit a new patient, which of your colleagues will you suggest as the best staff member to assign to make the home visit?
    1. An experienced and knowledgeable LPN who has worked for 10 years in home health.
    2. A respiratory therapist (RT) who regularly works with patients who are receiving home oxygen therapy.
    3. An RN who usually works in the maternal-child division of the public health agency.
    4. An on-call RN who works in the home health agency for a few days each month on an as-needed basis.

13. When you arrive at Mr. I.'s condominium, his wife answers the door and tells you that Mr. I. has been very lethargic and a little confused today. She says usually he is well-oriented and cheerful, in spite of his right-sided lung cancer diagnosis. Which information noted during your assessment is the best indicator that rapid nursing action is needed?
    1. The breath sounds are decreased on the right posterior chest.
    2. Mr. I. says that his appetite has not been very good recently.
    3. Mr. I.'s oral temperature is 101.0°F.
    4. The oral mucosa is pale and dry.

14. You call the oncologist to discuss Mr. I.'s condition and obtain an order to call an ambulance to transport him to the hospital ED for evaluation. Which information is most important to communicate when you call a report to the ED?
    1. Mr. I. has lung cancer and decreased breath sounds.
    2. Mr. I.'s assessment indicates probable dehydration.
    3. Mr. I. has an order for a CBC to be drawn today.
    4. Mr. I. is receiving chemotherapy and has a fever.

It is 12:30, and you are on your way to make your final visit of the day to Mr. D. The home health aide is just finishing his bath when you arrive and updates you with the patient's most recent vital signs and blood glucose:

Blood pressure	146/78
Pulse	88
Respiratory rate	24
Temperature	101.2°F
Blood glucose	326

15. Which of these assessment data requires nursing action most urgently?
    1. Blood pressure
    2. Glucose
    3. Respiratory rate
    4. Temperature

While you are assessing Mr. D., you change his left foot dressing and find that the wound on his left heel looks about the same as it did last week when you assessed it. It is dry-appearing and pale pink, with no wound drainage. When you ask him how the foot feels, he reminds you that he doesn't have much feeling because of his peripheral neuropathy.

You hear scattered coarse crackles and wheezes over the left posterior chest when you listen to his lung sounds. He says he feels short of breath with activity, but "My breathing is fine when I rest." He tells you that he has been coughing up some thick green mucus for the last few days. He has been voiding the usual amounts with no problems. His blood glucose levels have been in the 250 to 300 range for the last 2 days, but he has been using his sliding scale regular insulin as ordered. You check his oxygen saturation, which is 92% to 93%.

16. You call the physician to report Mr. D.'s status. What orders do you anticipate? (Choose all that apply.)
    1. Conduct urinalysis for culture and sensitivity.
    2. Obtain blood cultures from two separate sites.
    3. Obtain sputum specimen for Gram stain and culture.
    4. Swab wound and send for aerobic and anaerobic cultures.
    5. Administer ciprofloxacin (Cipro) 500 mg PO every 12 hours for 10 days.
    6. Check oxygen saturation daily.
    7. Transport patient to hospital via ambulance.
    8. Obtain and teach patient how to use incentive spirometer.
    9. Instruct patient to increase fluid intake to 2000 mL/day.

You plan to visit Mr. D. again early tomorrow and reassess his lung sounds, shortness of breath, temperature, and blood glucose level. After discussing Mr. D.'s plan of care with him and with the home health aide, you head back to your agency, where the mandatory in-service topic is how to prioritize care in the home health setting.

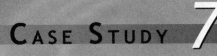

Spinal Cord Injury

Mr. M. is a 32-year-old man brought to the emergency department (ED) by paramedics after a fall from the second story roof of his home. He was placed on a spinal board to immobilize his spine. After spinal x-rays are obtained, the physicians determine that he has a vertical compression injury at the C4-5 level.

1. What is your priority concern at this time?
    1. Spinal immobilization to prevent additional injuries to the client
    2. Airway status due to interruption of spinal innervation to the respiratory muscles
    3. Potential for injuries related to the client's decreased perception of sensation
    4. Dysrhythmias due to disruption of the autonomic nervous system

2. Mr. M. is stabilized and moved to the neurologic intensive care unit with a diagnosis of spinal cord injury (SCI) at level C4-5. You are the admitting nurse and are working with an experienced nursing assistant. When performing frequent respiratory assessments, which action(s) can you delegate to the nursing assistant? (Choose all that apply.)
    1. Auscultate breath sounds every hour for decreased or absent ventilation.
    2. Ensure that oxygen is flowing at 5 L/minute via nasal cannula.
    3. Teach the client to breathe slowly and deeply and use incentive spirometry.
    4. Check the client's oxygen saturation by pulse oximetry every 2 hours.

3. An hour later, Mr. M.'s oxygen saturation drops to 88%, while his respirations are rapid and shallow. On auscultation, he has decreased breath sounds bilaterally. What is your best action at this time?
    1. Increase the oxygen flow to 10 L/minute.
    2. Suction the client for oral secretions.
    3. Notify the physician immediately.
    4. Call respiratory therapy for a non-rebreather mask.

After endotracheal intubation and placement on mechanical ventilation, Mr. M.'s oxygen saturation increases to 96%, and respirations decrease to 18 per minute (10 ventilator breaths per minute). On auscultation, he has breath sounds present in all lung lobes bilaterally.

4. The client's cervical injury has been immobilized with cervical tongs and traction to realign the vertebrae, facilitate bone healing, and prevent further injury. Which occurrence necessitates your immediate intervention?
   1. The traction weights are resting on the floor after the client is repositioned.
   2. The traction ropes are located within the pulley and hanging freely.
   3. The insertion sites for the cervical tongs are cleaned with hydrogen peroxide.
   4. The client is repositioned every 2 hours by using the log rolling technique.

5. Mr. M. has a nursing diagnosis of Ineffective Tissue Perfusion (spinal cord). What nursing action(s) should you delegate to the nursing student? (Choose all that apply.)
   1. Administer dantrolene (Dantrium) 25 mg orally to control muscle spasticity.
   2. Monitor traction ropes and weights while the client is repositioned.
   3. Check client's neurologic status for changes in movement and strength.
   4. Provide pin site care with hydrogen peroxide and normal saline.

6. Another diagnosis in Mr. M.'s nursing care plan is Impaired Physical Mobility. To prevent complications associated with this nursing diagnosis, which should you delegate to the experienced nursing assistant?
   1. Turn and reposition the client in bed every 2 hours.
   2. Inspect the client's skin for reddened areas.
   3. Perform range-of-motion (ROM) exercises every 8 hours.
   4. Administer enoxaparin (Lovenox) subcutaneously every 12 hours.

7. The nursing student asks how best to assess Mr. M's motor function. What is your best response?
   1. "Apply resistance while the client plantar flexes his feet."
   2. "Apply resistance while the client lifts his legs from the bed."
   3. "Apply downward pressure while the client shrugs his shoulders upward."
   4. "Make sure the client is able to grasp objects firmly and forms a fist."

8. Mr. M.'s condition has stabilized and he has been removed from the ventilator. His cervical injury is now immobilized with a halo fixation device and jacket. He has regained use of his arms and partial movement of his legs. Which instruction should you give to the nursing assistant providing assistance with activities of daily living?
   1. "Feed, bathe, and dress the client so that he does not become fatigued."
   2. "Encourage the client to perform all of his own self-care."
   3. "Allow the client to do what he can, then assist with what he can't."
   4. "Let the client's wife perform bathing and dressing actions."

9. Mr. M. continues to be incontinent. You plan to establish a bladder retraining program for him. Which of the following are important points for this program? (Choose all that apply.)
   1. Remove the indwelling Foley catheter.
   2. Use intermittent catheterization every 4 hours.
   3. Gradually increase intervals between catheterizations.
   4. Teach the client to initiate voiding by tapping on his bladder every 4 hours.
   5. Teach the client to perform self-catheterization if necessary.
   6. Administer bethanechol chloride (Urecholine) 20 mg orally twice a day.
   7. Encourage the client to limit fluid intake to 1000 mL of fluid every day.

10. Mr. M. is to be transferred to a rehabilitation facility. Which statement indicates that the client needs additional teaching?
    1. "After rehabilitation I may be able to achieve control of my bladder."
    2. "With rehabilitation I will regain all of my motor functions."
    3. "Rehabilitation will help me become as independent as possible."
    4. "After rehabilitation I hope to return to gainful employment."

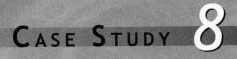

Multiple Patients with Adrenal Gland Disorders

Ms. B. was admitted through the emergency department (ED) after being hit in the abdomen by an automobile. An 18-gauge IV catheter was inserted in the left forearm, and normal saline was started at 100 mL/hr. The nursing assistant reports that her blood pressure has dropped to 92/58 and she is complaining of weakness, fatigue, and abdominal pain. When you assess Ms. B., you discover that she is also nauseated and has just vomited 560 mL.

Laboratory values from the ED:

Sodium	136 mEq/L
Potassium	3.7 mEq/L
Cortisol	2 mcg/dL (low)
Aldosterone	3 ng/dL (low)

1. What is your first action?
   1. Administer an anti-emetic.
   2. Measure abdominal girth.
   3. Notify the physician.
   4. Hang IV normal saline.

2. Ms. B.'s blood pressure is now 84/50. The physician's orders include the following. Which order will you implement first?
   1. Infuse normal saline at 250 mL/hour.
   2. Type and cross match for 2 units packed red blood cells.
   3. Insert second large-bore IV catheter.
   4. Administer prednisone 10 mg orally.

3. Which action(s) should you delegate to the nursing assistant, in providing care for Ms. B.? (Choose all that apply.)
   1. Encourage patient to take in adequate fluids.
   2. Take vital signs every 15 minutes.
   3. Record accurate intake and output every hour.
   4. Get a baseline weight to guide therapy.

4. Ms. B. develops diaphoresis, increased heart rate (124/minute), and tremors. She also complains of increasing headache. Which action should you take first?
    1. Check fingerstick glucose level.
    2. Check serum potassium level.
    3. Place patient on cardiac monitor.
    4. Decrease IV fluids to 100 mL/hour.

Ms. H. is admitted to the medical-surgical unit for a workup for Cushing's disease.

5. Which vital sign reported by the nursing assistant would be of most concern for a patient with Cushing's disease (hypercortisolism)?
    1. Heart rate 102 beats/minute
    2. Respiratory rate 26/minute
    3. Blood pressure 156/88
    4. Oral temperature 101.8°F

6. Which factor reported by Ms. H. supports the diagnosis of Cushing's disease?
    1. Cessation of menses at age 33
    2. Increased craving for salty foods
    3. Weight loss of 25 pounds
    4. Nausea, diarrhea, loss of appetite

7. A student nurse will assess Ms. H. What findings will you teach the student nurse to expect if a patient has Cushing's disease? (Choose all that apply.)
    1. Truncal obesity
    2. Weight loss
    3. Bruising
    4. Poor healing

8. Ms H. is given the diagnosis of Cushing's disease due to increased secretion of adrenocorticotropic hormone (ACTH) and is scheduled for adrenalectomy. Which preoperative action(s) should you delegate to the LPN/LVN? (Choose all that apply.)
    1. Assess patient's cardiac rhythm.
    2. Review patient's laboratory results.
    3. Check fingerstick glucose results.
    4. Administer sliding scale insulin.

9. Ms. H. has a nursing diagnosis of Risk for Infection related to immunosuppression and inadequate primary defenses. Which nursing care action(s) should you delegate to the nursing assistant? (Choose all that apply.)
    1. Provide patient with a soft toothbrush and electric razor.
    2. Instruct patient to avoid activities that can result in skin trauma.
    3. Remind patient to change positions in bed every 2 hours.
    4. Monitor patient's skin for reddened areas, excoriation, and edema.

10. Ms. H. has had a complete adrenalectomy, and you are preparing to educate her about cortisol replacement therapy. Which key points will you include in the teaching plan? (Choose all that apply.)
    1. "Take your medication in divided doses: first dose in the morning, second dose between 4 and 6 PM."
    2. "Take your medications on an empty stomach to facilitate absorption."
    3. "Weigh yourself daily using the same scale and wearing the same amount of clothes."
    4. "Never skip a dose of medication."
    5. "Call your doctor if you experience persistent nausea, severe diarrhea, or fever."
    6. "Report any rapid weight gain, round face, fluid retention, or swelling to your doctor."

11. You are admitting a patient with the diagnosis of primary hyperaldosteronism (Conn's syndrome). Which laboratory value is of most concern?
    1. Serum calcium
    2. Serum sodium
    3. Serum potassium
    4. Serum creatinine

Ms. L. is a 59-year-old woman admitted for intermittent episodes of high blood pressure who experiences headaches, diaphoresis, and chest pain. She says that she gets frightened and feels a "sense of doom" when these episodes occur. The endocrinologist's preliminary diagnosis is rule out pheochromocytoma.

12. What assessment technique should you avoid when admitting Ms. L.?
    1. Abdominal palpation
    2. Extremity reflex checks
    3. Pupillary reaction to light
    4. Stand for baseline weight

13. The physician orders a 24-hour urine collection for vanillylmandelic acid (VMA), metanephrine, and catecholamines. For which instruction given to Ms. L. by the nursing student should you intervene?
    1. "You will be on a special diet for 2 to 3 days before the urine collection for this test."
    2. "You should not drink caffeinated beverages or eat citrus fruits, bananas, or chocolate."
    3. "You will remain on your usual medication regimen including your aspirin and the beta blocker for your high blood pressure."
    4. "In 2 to 3 days you will begin to collect the 24-hour urine after discarding the first void in the morning."

14. When providing nursing care for Ms. L., which action should you delegate to the nursing assistant?
    1. Work with the patient to identify stressful situations that may lead to a hypertensive crisis.
    2. Remind the patient not to smoke, drink caffeinated beverages, or change positions suddenly.
    3. Monitor the patient's hydration status and report manifestations of dehydration or fluid overload.
    4. Tell the patient to limit activity and remain in a calm, restful environment during headaches

15. As charge nurse, which patient(s) will you assign to the new graduate nurse who has just completed orientation to the unit? (Choose all that apply.)
    1. Ms. L. with pheochromocytoma, who is scheduled for adrenalectomy and needs pre-operative teaching
    2. Ms. B. with adrenal gland hypofunction, whose blood pressure is dropping and is experiencing an Addisonian crisis
    3. Ms. H. with Cushing's disease, who is very anxious and fearful about her scheduled adrenal surgery
    4. Mr. J. with hyperaldosteronism, whose current serum potassium level is 3.2 mEq/L

Multiple Clients with Gastrointestinal Problems

You are the team leader caring for six gastrointestinal (GI) clients on a medical-surgical unit. The team includes a new graduate RN, who has recently completed hospital orientation, and an experienced nursing assistant. The clients are as follows:

- *Ms. H., a 36-year-old woman with right upper quadrant (RUQ) pain that radiates to the right shoulder. She has a history of gallstones. She was admitted through the emergency department (ED) last night for acute cholecystitis. Night shift reports, "She had a good night."*
- *Mr. R., a 57-year-old man with umbilical pain. Pain is described as 7/10 despite medication, and radiates to the back. Mr. R. was admitted with acute pancreatitis. He is NPO (nothing by mouth) with a nasogastric (NG) tube and IV. "He's been anxious and belligerent." White blood cell count (WBC) and blood glucose are increased.*
- *Ms. D., a 60-year-old woman receiving IV antibiotics every 6 hours. She has an NG tube in place that will probably be removed tomorrow. She reports dull but continuous left lower quadrant (LLQ) pain. She has a history of alternating diarrhea and constipation. Last night she reported constipation but no other complaints.*
- *Mr. A., a 26-year-old man, will be discharged in the afternoon. He had discharge teaching from the enterostomal therapist yesterday regarding his infected wound secondary to a ruptured appendix; he wants a review of the wound care instructions before he leaves.*
- *Ms. T., a 29-year-old woman, appears wasted and malnourished. She has severe diarrhea and reports pre-defecation abdominal pain and generalized tenderness to palpation. She is receiving total parenteral nutrition (TPN) through a central line.*
- *Mr. K., an 85-year-old man, is frail but alert and oriented. He was transferred from an extended-care facility for a percutaneous endoscopic gastrostomy (PEG) that was placed 5 days ago. He has a large family. They ask a lot of questions and argue continuously amongst themselves and with the staff. His vital signs are stable.*

1. Which client(s) can be assigned to the new RN? (Choose all that apply.)
    1. Ms. H.
    2. Mr. R.
    3. Ms. D.
    4. Mr. A.
    5. Ms. T.
    6. Mr. K.

2. The night nurse gives a brief and incomplete report. Which question should you pose to the night shift nurse to help determine the priority actions for Ms. H.?
   1. "What are her vital signs?"
   2. "Is she going to OR or Radiology this morning?"
   3. "Is she still having pain?"
   4. "Does she need any morning medications?"

3. Prioritize the order for assessing these clients.
   1. Mr. R.
   2. Ms. D.
   3. Ms. T.
   4. Mr. A.

   ____, ____, ____, ____

4. The clients must receive their routine morning medications. Which client should receive his or her medication last?
   1. Mr. K.
   2. Mr. A.
   3. Ms. H.
   4. Ms. D.

5. Which task(s) should you delegate to the nursing assistant? (Choose all that apply.)
   1. Assist Ms. T. with perineal care after diarrheal episodes.
   2. Take vital signs every 2 hours for Mr. R.
   3. Transport Ms. H. to the radiology department.
   4. Gently cleanse nares around Ms. D.'s NG tube.
   5. Take dressing materials to Mr. A's room.

6. Which reporting task(s) is (are) appropriate to delegate to the nursing assistant? (Choose all that apply.)
   1. Assess for perianal excoriation when cleaning Ms. T.
   2. Report the quality and color of NG drainage for Ms. D.
   3. Report if Mr. L.'s BP <100/60 or pulse >110/minute.
   4. Report if any of the clients complain of pain.

7. What would be the first choice of medication for Mr. R.'s severe pancreatic pain?
   1. meperidine (Demerol)
   2. morphine sulfate
   3. acetaminophen and hydrocodone bitartrate (Lortab)
   4. acetaminophen and propoxyphene napsylate (Darvocet)

8. Ms. H.'s doctor told her that she would probably need a laparoscopic cholecystectomy; however, the hepatobiliary iminodiacetic acid (HIDA) scan and laboratory results are still pending. Ms. H. asks, "What should I expect?" What is the best intervention at this point?
   1. Describe the surgical procedure.
   2. Call the physician to come and speak with her.
   3. Provide some written material about gallbladder (GB) disease and options.
   4. Demonstrate coughing and deep breathing exercises.

9. Ms. T. is discouraged and dispirited about her ulcerative colitis. She is resistant to TPN because "I'm being kept alive with tubes." Which explanation will encourage Ms. T. to continue with the TPN therapy?
   1. "It will help you regain your weight."
   2. "It will create a positive nitrogen balance."
   3. "Your doctor has ordered this important therapy for you."
   4. "Your bowel can rest and the diarrhea will decrease."

10. Ms. T. is on sulfasalazine (Azulfidine) 500 mg PO every 6 hours. Which assessment finding concerns you the most?
    1. Urine discoloration
    2. Nausea and vomiting
    3. Decreased urine output
    4. Headache

11. The nursing assistant asks, "Why can't Ms. T. get out of bed and do things for herself? She's only 29." What is your best response?
    1. "The doctor ordered bedrest for a few days."
    2. "She is too depressed and malnourished."
    3. "Acute exacerbations require decreased GI motility."
    4. "Decreased activity helps decrease the diarrhea."

12. You are teaching the new nurse about enteral feedings for clients such as Mr. K. In the postoperative period, when can enteral feedings be started?
    1. Within 6–8 hours after the procedure
    2. When bowel sounds are present, usually within 24 hours
    3. When the client complains of feeling hungry
    4. On a schedule determined by the pharmacy

13. Because of Mr. K.'s advanced age, which complication(s) of enteral feedings may occur? (Choose all that apply.)
    1. Hyperglycemia
    2. Hypertension
    3. Aspiration
    4. Diarrhea

14. During the midmorning, several events happen at the same time. Prioritize the order that you will attend to these issues, either personally or by delegation. (Each number may be used more than once as you make decisions about prioritization and delegation.)
    1. Ms D. has accidentally pulled out her IV lock.
    2. Ms. H. calls for an antiemetic for vomiting bile.
    3. Mr. R. is walking down the hall, threatening to leave.
    4. Mr. K.'s family wants to speak to the doctor.

    ____, ____, ____, ____, ____

15. After lunch, you find the new RN in the bathroom crying. She tells you, "I'm a terrible nurse. I am so disorganized and so far behind. I'm going to quit. I hate this job." What is the best thing to do?
    1. Send her on a break off the unit.
    2. Offer to take one of her clients.
    3. Ask the nursing assistant to help her.
    4. Calm her down and help her prioritize.

16. Mr. A. reluctantly discloses to you that his financial and social situations are problematic. Which aspect of his situation has the most impact on the discharge teaching?
    1. He is homeless and has no family in the city.
    2. He has no money for the prescribed medications.
    3. He has no transportation to the follow-up appointment.
    4. He cannot read or write very well.

17. While you are teaching Mr. A. about dressing changes, he tells you, "When you live on the street, you can't do everything the way you nurses do in the hospital." What is the most important thing to emphasize in helping him to accomplish self-care?
    1. Use new sterile gloves every time.
    2. Maintain a sterile field for supplies.
    3. Wash your hands before dressing change.
    4. Discard any opened packages of 4 × 4.

18. What information regarding Mr. R. is appropriate to report to the physician? (Choose all that apply.)
    1. HCT is decreased >10%.
    2. Calcium is <1.9 mmol.
    3. Po_2 is <60 mm Hg.
    4. Pain is unrelieved by medication.

19. The physician has been paged and is en route to see Mr. R. The client is increasingly agitated and confused. He pulls out his IV and NG tube. His skin is pale and clammy. Pulse 120/min, BP 140/60. Prioritize the steps in caring for Mr. R.
    1. Restart the IV.
    2. Place the pulse oximeter.
    3. Stay with the client.
    4. Give supplemental oxygen.
    5. Have colleague gather equipment.
    6. Check blood sugar.
    7. Repeat vital signs.

    ＿＿, ＿＿, ＿＿, ＿＿, ＿＿, ＿＿, ＿＿

20. The physician arrives while you are caring for Mr. R. Based on Mr. R.'s change of status (refer to questions 18 and 19), what physician order do you anticipate?
    1. Obtain additional labs and an ECG, and apply restraints.
    2. Prepare Mr. R. for emergency surgery.
    3. Prepare Mr. R. for transfer to the ICU.
    4. Reestablish the IV, NG, etc., and keep him/her informed.

21. What tasks should be accomplished toward the end of the shift before leaving for the day? (Choose all that apply.)
    1. Complete documentation on all assigned clients.
    2. Admit a new client from the ED.
    3. Check all IV sites and total IV fluids.
    4. Ask the assistant to obtain repeat vital signs on all clients.
    5. Briefly check and assess every client.
    6. Thank ancillary staff for their help.
    7. Complete Mr. R.'s transfer to the intensive care unit.

Multiple Patients with Pain

You are the team leader caring for patients on a medical-surgical unit. The team includes a new graduate RN, who has recently completed hospital orientation, and a nursing assistant. Your patients are listed below:

- *Ms. R., a 55-year-old woman with rheumatoid arthritis, is 1 day post-operative for shoulder arthroplasty. She reports morning stiffness in her joints. Swelling is noted in bilateral wrists and proximal interphalangeal (PIP) joints. She has been using patient-controlled analgesia (PCA) morphine with relief.*
- *Mr. L., a 35-year-old man with a history of kidney stones, reports severe back and flank pain intermittently (3–8/10). Night shift reports episodic nausea and vomiting with hematuria and dysuria. Mr. L. was admitted through the emergency department (ED) at 22:00. He is on a PCA pump.*
- *Mr. H., a 28-year-old man, is currently in the operating room (OR) for an inguinal hernia repair. He should return from the OR later in the shift.*
- *Mr. O., an 18-year-old man, sustained a right tibial-fibula fracture in a motorcycle accident 7 hours ago. He has extensive road rash underneath the cast and on the right anterior-lateral body. Although initial chest and abdominal trauma were ruled out in ED, he is being monitored for occult trauma.*
- *Ms. J., a 65-year-old woman with end-stage multiple myeloma, is receiving palliative pain management; the family is considering hospice care. She has been on the unit for 2 weeks. Her physician signed the do-not-resuscitate (DNR) order 3 days ago.*
- *Mr. A., a 40-year-old man, has been on the unit for 3 weeks. He is receiving IV antibiotics for bacterial pneumonia. He has a history of IV drug abuse and is positive for human immunodeficiency virus (HIV). Mr. A.'s condition was deteriorating during the night shift.*

1. You decide to do a brief round on all the patients prior to shift report, for safety and to help determine acuity and assignments. List the priority order to briefly check in on these patients.
   1. Ms. R.
   2. Mr. L.
   3. Mr. H.
   4. Mr. O.
   5. Ms. J.
   6. Mr. A.

   ____, ____, ____, ____, ____, ____

2. Which of the six patient(s) can be assigned to the new RN? (Choose all that apply.)
   1. Ms. R.
   2. Mr. L.
   3. Mr. H.
   4. Mr. O.
   5. Ms. J.
   6. Mr. A.

3. The new nurse tells you that she cannot find any documentation that shows Mr. L.'s last dose of pain medication. What action should occur first?
   1. Help the new nurse look at the chart and MAR.
   2. Tell the new nurse to ask the night nurse before she leaves.
   3. You should speak to the night shift nurse about the documentation.
   4. Have the new nurse ask Mr. L. when he last had medication.

4. Which morning task(s) can be delegated to the nursing assistant? (Choose all that apply.)
   1. Assist Ms. R. with morning care.
   2. Reinforce to Mr. L. to save urine for straining.
   3. Prepare Mr. H.'s room for return from the OR.
   4. Start Mr. O.'s skin hygiene.
   5. Get coffee for Ms. J.'s family.

5. Which task(s) related to pain management can you delegate to the nursing assistant? (Choose all that apply.)
   1. Report on grimacing seen in unresponsive patients.
   2. Ask about the location, quality, and radiation of pain.
   3. Remind the patients to report pain as necessary.
   4. Observe for relief after medication is given.
   5. Ask patients directly, "Are you having pain?"

6. For Mr. O., in addition to pain medication, which action will help the most to relieve pain associated with the tibula-fibula fracture?
   1. Instruct him to periodically move toes.
   2. Use diversional therapy.
   3. Elevate leg above the heart.
   4. Place him in high-Fowler's position.

7. Mr. O. is at risk for compartment syndrome because of the cast. Which pain assessment would alert you to compartment syndrome?
   1. Pain on passive motion
   2. Sudden increase in pain
   3. Pain with dorsiflexion of the foot
   4. Pain-free despite no recent medication

8. Mr. L. calls for pain medication. He describes the pain as "the worst pain I have ever had." He is crying, diaphoretic, and pacing around the room. What is your priority action?
   1. Instruct Mr. L. to do deep breathing exercises.
   2. Remind Mr. L. to use the PCA pump.
   3. Give him a PRN IV bolus dose as ordered.
   4. Call the physician immediately.

9. Mr. H. returns from the OR. He says that he is "afraid to walk because it will make the pain really bad." What will you explain as being the best option?
    1. Pain medication every 4 hours if he needs it
    2. Medication 45 minutes before ambulation or dressing changes
    3. Around-the-clock pain medication even if he has no complaints
    4. To talk to the physician for reassurance about the treatment plan

10. During the shift, several events occur at the same time. Prioritize the order for addressing these problems, either personally or by delegation. (Each number may be used more than once as you make decisions about prioritization and delegation.)
    1. Mr. L. is calling out loudly about his right flank pain (9/10).
    2. Ms. J.'s PCA pump is accidentally pushed over and "broken."
    3. Another nurse needs narcotics wastage witnessed.
    4. Mr. A. is urinating in the corner of his room.

    _____, _____, _____, _____, _____, _____

11. One of the staff members is talking about Mr. A. in the medication room. "He complains all the time about pain everywhere. Well, he is going to have pain. He's a drug addict, what does he expect?" What is your best response to this comment?
    1. "All patients have a right to care regardless of race, creed, etc."
    2. "I'll take Mr. A., I don't mind taking care of him."
    3. "You should talk to the supervisor about this."
    4. "What can we do to help Mr. A, so he complains less?"

12. Which team members (RN, nursing assistant, physical therapist) should perform the tasks related to Mr. A.'s pain management?

    1. Instruct and supervise the transcutaneous electrical nerve stimulation (TENS) unit. _____

    2. Administer non-opioid pain medication. _____

    3. Answer questions about medication side effects._____

    4. Perform ultrasound treatments. _____

    5. Suggest that relatives bring personal comfort items. _____

    6. Assist the patient to change position every 2 hours. _____

13. Mr. H. is given a dose of pain medication. One hour later he is anxious and appears uncomfortable and asks, "What's the matter? Is something wrong? I'm still hurting." What action should you take first?
    1. Call the physician for a change in medication or dose.
    2. Keep the patient NPO in case he has to go back to surgery.
    3. Check for bladder distention and last voiding.
    4. Reassure the patient that the hernia is not recurring.

14. Mr. L. reports that the pain has decreased compared to earlier but now he is having dysuria and other symptoms. Which symptom is the greatest concern?
    1. Painless hematuria with small clots
    2. Dull pain that radiates into the genitalia
    3. Pain-free, but scant output
    4. Sensation of urinary urgency

15. The nursing assistant reports that the new nurse is undermedicating the patients. What is the best way to handle this situation?
    1. Ignore her; she is not qualified to judge an RN.
    2. Ask the assistant to give specific examples.
    3. Go to the new nurse and question her.
    4. Do an assessment on all of the nurse's patients.

16. Ms. J. is receiving continuous opiates to control her pain. Which side effect occurring on your shift is your major concern?
    1. Constipation
    2. Respiratory depression
    3. Nausea and vomiting
    4. Sedation

17. Ms. J. is having severe pain and admits to it; however, she becomes very anxious when certain family members come and go and refuses to take the pain medication. Which adjunct medication would be most useful to Ms. J. to help her manage these episodes?
    1. naproxen sodium (Naprosyn)
    2. doxepin hydrochloride (Sinequan)
    3. lorazepam (Ativan)
    4. dicyclomine hydrochloride (Bentyl)

18. Ms. J.'s son repeatedly insists that Ms. J. is not getting enough pain medication. He threatens to sue. You have used therapeutic communication skills with the son and advocated for the patient with the physician. The physician informs you, "I'll be in tomorrow. Just tell the son to chill out." What is your best action?
    1. Call another physician.
    2. Continue to use the current orders.
    3. Have the son call the physician.
    4. Notify the unit manager.

19. It is the end of the shift, and the new nurse is trying to give pain medication to one patient, provide comfort measures for another patient, and redo pain assessments on all her patients. Her documentation is incomplete. What should you do?
    1. Offer to help her by performing the comfort measures.
    2. Let her struggle through so she can find her own way.
    3. Help her to prioritize and delegate the tasks.
    4. Ask someone from the oncoming shift to help her.

Multiple Clients with Cancer

You are the team leader caring for clients on a medical-surgical oncology unit. The team includes an experienced chemotherapy-certified RN, a new nursing assistant, and a first-semester nursing student. Your patients are listed below:

- *Mr. L., a 50-year-old man, was transferred 2 days ago from the surgical intensive care unit (SICU) following a tracheostomy and partial laryngectomy. He has a nasogastric (NG) tube and a tracheostomy tube and is currently receiving chemotherapy. He received radiation therapy prior to surgery.*
- *Mr. N., a 68-year-old man, presented to his physician with fever, weight loss, and painless axillary nodes. Following a lymph node biopsy, he was diagnosed with non-Hodgkin's lymphoma. He is receiving chemotherapy and is on neutropenic precautions. He currently is afebrile, in good spirits, and feels reasonably well.*
- *Mr. B., a 59-year-old man, presented to his doctor with painless hematuria and was subsequently diagnosed with bladder cancer. He was admitted for intravesical chemotherapy. He received procedural teaching prior to admission. He is alert, conversant, and independently performing activities of daily living (ADLs).*
- *Ms. C., a 70-year-old woman, went to her doctor for rectal bleeding and a change in bowel habits. She is 5 days post-operative for a bowel resection and colostomy. She is progressing well, but needs and likes companionship at the bedside.*
- *Mr. U., a 62-year-old man with a history of cough, hemoptysis, fatigue, and dyspnea, underwent bronchoscopy and sputum cytology and was diagnosed with non–small-cell lung cancer. He is 1 day postoperative for pulmonary resection and has a chest tube drainage system.*
- *Ms. G., a 65-year-old woman, was admitted for a right breast lumpectomy scheduled for later in the day, which will be followed by radiation therapy. She appears nervous and tearful and is frequently asking questions.*

1. You make very brief rounds on each client prior to receiving shift report to ensure safety and to help you determine assignments. What will these brief assessments entail? (Choose all that apply.)
   1. Ask, "How are you feeling?"
   2. Note mental status (alert and oriented?).
   3. Take vital signs and look at intake and output (I&O).
   4. Palpate chest/abdominal areas for pain.
   5. Note presence and complexity of equipment.
   6. Note ease of respiratory effort.

2. The first-semester nursing student tells you that her clinical assignment for the day is to take vital signs and to do a client history that will take about 1 or 2 hours to complete. Which client(s) would you recommend she approach to fulfill her assignment? (Choose all that apply.)
   1. Mr. L.
   2. Mr. N.
   3. Mr. B.
   4. Ms. C.
   5. Mr. U.
   6. Ms. G.

3. You must assign a nursing assistant to help care for Mr. N. For this neutropenic client, which factor has the most impact in assigning a nursing assistant?
   1. Nursing assistant is in the first trimester of pregnancy.
   2. Nursing assistant has had cold symptoms for 3 days.
   3. Nursing assistant has no experience with neutropenic precautions.
   4. Nursing assistant has generalized fear of isolation clients.

4. In the early post-operative period, what is the priority nursing diagnosis for Mr. L.?
   1. Risk for Infection related to chemotherapy and surgical procedure
   2. Impaired Nutrition related to pre-surgical dysphagia and malignancy
   3. Impaired Communication related to tracheostomy tube
   4. Risk for Aspiration related to secretions and removal of epiglottis

5. What assessment finding for Mr. L. should be reported to the physician?
   1. Frank bleeding from the tracheostomy site
   2. Increased secretions in/around the tracheostomy tube
   3. Inability to swallow own saliva
   4. Coughing up secretions

6. Clients receiving chemotherapy are at risk for thrombocytopenia related to chemotherapy or disease processes. What actions are needed for clients who must be placed on bleeding precautions? (Choose all that apply.)
   1. Provide mouthwash with alcohol for oral rinse.
   2. Use paper tape on fragile skin.
   3. Provide a soft toothbrush or oral sponge.
   4. Lubricate rectal suppositories.
   5. Avoid aspirin or aspirin-containing products.
   6. Avoid overinflation of blood pressure cuffs.
   7. Pad sharp corners of furniture.

7. Mr. B. will receive an intravesical chemotherapy, bacillus Calmette-Guérin (BCG) instillation. Place the steps in correct order.
   1. Clamp the catheter.
   2. Insert a Foley catheter.
   3. Instill BCG fluid via catheter.
   4. Change position side to side every 15 minutes for 2 hours.
   5. Direct client to drink two glasses of water to flush the bladder.
   6. Unclamp the catheter at the end of 2 hours.

   _____, _____, _____, _____, _____, _____

8. You delegate disposal of Mr. B.'s Foley bag and fluid contents to the nursing assistant. What special instructions should you give?
    1. No special handling of the bag or contents is required.
    2. "Wear a lead apron when emptying the Foley."
    3. "Disinfect the toilet with bleach for 6 hours after treatment."
    4. "Wear sterile gloves when handling the bag and contents."

9. If normal voiding does not resume after removal of Mr. B.'s catheter, when should you notify the physician?
    1. Within 6 hours
    2. Within 24 hours
    3. Within 3 days
    4. Within 1 week

10. During the midmorning, several events occur at the same time. Prioritize the events in the order that they should be delegated or addressed.
    1. Mr. B. complains of dysuria.
    2. Mr. U.'s chest drainage system tips over.
    3. Mr. N. has a fever of 101°F.
    4. Mr. L.'s trach tube needs to be suctioned.
    5. Ms. C. has a swollen, tender, red calf.

    _____, _____, _____, _____, _____

11. The nursing student tearfully reports to you, "I took some flowers into Mr. N.'s room to cheer him up and he told me that he didn't think he was supposed to have flowers. I took them out of the room right away and then I realized I had made a mistake." What should you do first?
    1. Direct the student to read the isolation precautions before entering the room.
    2. Call the nursing instructor and report the student for making an error.
    3. Acknowledge and praise the student for taking responsibility for the mistake.
    4. Write an incident report and have the student and instructor sign it.

12. In preparing a client like Ms. C. for her bowel surgery, which team member (RN, nursing assistant, enterostomal therapist) under the appropriate supervision should be assigned to each of these actions?
    1. Assist Ms. C. with bowel evacuation. _____
    2. Administer sulfonamides by mouth. _____
    3. Explain the need for a rectal dressing. _____
    4. Answer questions about ostomy. _____
    5. Advise about optimal stoma placement. _____

13. Several days after surgery, Ms. C. repeatedly refuses to perform a return demonstration of any aspect of colostomy care. Despite steady improvement and independent resumption of other ADLs, she protests, "I'm too weak. You'll have to do it for me." What is the priority diagnosis for Ms. C.?
    1. Activity Intolerance related to disease process
    2. Risk for Impaired Tissue Integrity related to ostomy
    3. Knowledge Deficit related to procedure
    4. Coping, Defensive related to change in health and ADL

14. The nursing staff is making suggestions about how to help Ms. C. deal with the colostomy care. Which suggestion will you try first?
    1. Verbally re-explain the procedure and give her written material.
    2. Have a family member come in and do it for her.
    3. Continue to do it for her until she is ready.
    4. Ask her to hold the clamp while the bag is being emptied.

15. During pre-operative teaching, Ms. G. begins to cry and asks, "What do you think about this breast surgery? My friend's arm got really swollen after she had the surgery. Can't I just take medication?" What is the priority diagnosis for Ms. G?
    1. Anxiety related to unknown outcomes
    2. Disturbed Body Image related to imminent loss of body part
    3. Knowledge Deficit related to treatment plan
    4. Noncompliance related to surgical procedure

16. Which assessment finding is the most critical?
    1. Mr. U. has tracheal deviation.
    2. Mr. L.'s trach tube is pulsating.
    3. Mr. N. is having dysrhythmias.
    4. Ms. C. has severe abdominal pain.

17. List three additional assessment findings of tension pneumothorax that help you identify this potentially life-threatening emergency.

    _____

    _____

    _____

18. You determine that Mr. U. has developed a tension pneumothorax. He is currently receiving high-flow oxygen. What is the priority action?
    1. Remove the occlusive dressing around the chest wound.
    2. Perform a needle thoracotomy with a 14- to 16-gauge catheter needle.
    3. Initiate cardiopulmonary resuscitation (CPR).
    4. Call for the crash cart and intubation equipment.

Gastrointestinal Bleeding

Mr. S., a 50-year-old white man, drove himself to the emergency department (ED) after vomiting bright red blood twice within 6 hours. He arrives alert and oriented but appears anxious. He is a vague historian, but admits to drinking "a few" last weekend. He knows that he is "supposed to stop drinking" and takes "something for his stomach," but he cannot recall the name of the medication. He complains of intermittent dizziness and fatigue that has been worsening over the past 2 days. Skin is dry and pale. Abdomen is slightly distended. He reports pain (4/10) in the mid-epigastric area. Capillary refill is >3 seconds, BP is 140/90, pulse is 110/minute, respirations are 24/minute, and temperature is 37.2°C.

1. What is the priority nursing diagnosis for Mr. S.?
   1. Risk of Aspiration related to active bleeding
   2. Anxiety related to uncertainty of health status
   3. Deficient Fluid Volume related to vomiting blood and gastric secretions
   4. Noncompliance related to alcohol consumption and medication

2. What actions are appropriate in the care of this patient? (Choose all that apply.)
   1. Start a peripheral IV using a 22-gauge catheter.
   2. Initiate I&O with hourly urine output measurements.
   3. Check emesis and stool for occult blood.
   4. Monitor hemoglobin and hematocrit every 4 hours.
   5. Maintain the patient in a semi- or high-Fowler's position.
   6. Prepare the patient for surgery.

3. Which task is appropriate to assign to the nursing assistant?
   1. Obtain repeat vital signs every 2 hours.
   2. Gather equipment for nasogastric lavage.
   3. Check the blood glucose level every 2 hours.
   4. Notify the family (with patient's permission).

4. The physician has ordered several STAT interventions for Mr. S. To complete these interventions in a rapid and efficient manner, you ask several team members to assist. Which staff member under the supervision of an RN (nursing assistant, paramedic, RN, clergy, LPN/LVN) will you delegate to perform each task?

   1. Place an automatic BP cuff. _____

   2. Establish two peripheral IVs with 16-gauge catheters._____

   3. Place an NG tube and initiate saline lavage._____

   4. Insert a Foley catheter attached to a urinometer. _____

   5. Set up blood transfusion equipment. _____

   6. Liaison with family members in the waiting room. _____

   7. Assess baseline breath and bowel sounds. _____

5. You are performing additional assessment and history on Mr. S. Which finding should you immediately report to the physician?
   1. Melena stools
   2. History of NSAID use
   3. Tense rigid abdomen
   4. Probable HIV+ status

6. The physician orders a nasogastric (NG) tube insertion with saline lavage. List the correct order of actions for this procedure.
   1. Measure tube from tip of nose, to earlobe, to xiphoid process.
   2. Place the patient in a high-Fowler's position.
   3. Ask the patient to sip water as you pass the tube.
   4. Have the patient bend the chin forward.
   5. Auscultate and check pH to verify tube placement.
   6. Inspect for patient's most patent nostril.
   7. Insert the tube into the most patent nostril.

   _____, _____, _____, _____, _____, _____, _____

7. Despite your best efforts at therapeutic communication, Mr. S. refuses to cooperate with the NG tube insertion. He threatens to leave "if you stick that tube down my nose again." What should you do first?
   1. Physically restrain him and insert the tube.
   2. Explain the AMA (against medical advice) form.
   3. Notify the nursing supervisor and patient advocate.
   4. Page the physician and document the attempt.

8. You discover that the phlebotomist drew the STAT blood work from another patient, not Mr. S. What should you do first?
   1. Call the phlebotomist to come back.
   2. Draw the blood sample yourself.
   3. Report the phlebotomist to his supervisor.
   4. Ask the phlebotomist to explain what happened.

9. The physician orders a STAT blood transfusion. In the event of an emergency, for a patient such as Mr. S., a type-specific un–cross-matched blood could be used. What do you anticipate as the blood product in this case?
   1. O negative
   2. AB negative
   3. AB positive
   4. A negative

10. You are preparing to administer a blood transfusion to Mr. S. Place the steps of transfusion in the appropriate order.
    1. Prime the correct tubing and filter with normal saline.
    2. Take the vital signs before starting the transfusion.
    3. Transfuse the first 50 mL slowly; monitor closely.
    4. Inspect the bag for leaks, clots, or unusual color.
    5. Compare the bag label with the chart and blood bank forms.
    6. Two nurses (or MDs) compare ID blood band with tag on blood bag.
    7. Repeat vital signs after 15 minutes and then every hour until complete.
    8. Document outcomes, names of personnel, and starting/ending times.

    ____, ____, ____, ____, ____, ____, ____, ____

11. What medication is the physician most likely to order for emergency treatment of acute and severe bleeding of Mr. S.'s ulcer?
    1. Antacid
    2. Histamine H_2-receptor antagonist
    3. Vasopressin
    4. Proton pump inhibitor

Head and Leg Trauma and Shock

Ms. A. is a 20-year-old college student who had been drinking at a fraternity party before she fell from a second-floor balcony. Paramedics were called by one of the more sober students at the party and Ms. A. has just arrived in the emergency department (ED). A fellow college student who accompanies Ms. A. tells you that she was "completely knocked out right after the fall. But then, she woke up a little, so we thought she was okay—until she stopped moving again."

You are assigned as the ED triage nurse. When you assess Ms. A., there is no response to commands or to having her name called. She extends her arms and legs stiffly when nailbed pressure is applied, but there is still no verbal response. Her eyes are shut and she does not open them even with the nailbed pressure. When you open her eyelids, you see that her pupils are unequal, with the right pupil larger than the left. The pupil response when you shine a flashlight into her eyes is sluggish.

Ms. A.'s blood pressure (BP) is 70/30, she is in a sinus bradycardia with a rate of 40, and her respiratory rate is 6 breaths per minute. Her respirations are irregular and she has 20-second periods of apnea. You note a large occipital laceration and her left leg is misaligned.

The paramedics have a cervical collar and backboard in place. She has a 16-gauge Abocath inserted at the left antecubital area and lactated Ringer's solution is infusing at 150 mL/hour.

1. Which additional assessment is most important to obtain at this time?
   1. Temperature
   2. Breath sounds
   3. Pedal pulses
   4. O_2 saturation

2. What is the best way to clearly document Ms. A.'s level of consciousness (LOC)?
   1. Client has a decreased LOC.
   2. Client is unresponsive.
   3. Client Glasgow Coma Scale = 4.
   4. Client is comatose.

3. When describing Ms. A.'s neurologic assessment, you will chart "Client demonstrates _____ posturing in response to nailbed pressure."

4. Based on Ms. A.'s vital signs, she appears to be in shock. Which type(s) of shock are you most concerned about for this client? (Choose all that apply.)
   1. Cardiogenic
   2. Hypovolemic
   3. Neurogenic
   4. Septic
   5. Anaphylactic

5. You are working with Dr. G., a new medical resident whose first day in the ED rotation is today. Which action by Dr. G. will require you to intervene immediately?
   1. Dr. G. assesses for Babinski's sign.
   2. Dr. G increases the IV rate to 200 mL/hour.
   3. Dr. G. orders a STAT electrocardiogram.
   4. Dr. G. prepares to do a lumbar puncture.

6. After triaging Ms. A., you need to assign one of your ED staff members to care for her. Which of these staff members will be most appropriate to assign to take primary responsibility for Ms. A.'s ongoing care?
   1. A temporary agency RN with extensive previous ED experience, who has been in your ED for 3 days
   2. An LPN with 10 years of experience in your ED, who is in the last semester of an RN program
   3. An RN who has worked in your ED for the last 5 years after transferring from the mother-baby unit
   4. An RN who has 12 years of experience in the intensive care unit (ICU) and has been floated to the ED today

7. Ms. A. suddenly begins to vomit. Which action should the nurse take first?
   1. Utilize the backboard to logroll Ms. A. to her side.
   2. Suction Ms. A.'s airway with a Yankauer suction device.
   3. Hyperoxygenate Ms. A. with a bag-valve-mask system.
   4. Insert nasogastric (NG) tube and connect to low suction.

Laboratory tests that were drawn when Ms. A. arrived in the ED are faxed to the RN. CBC results are:

Hemoglobin 12.6 g/dL
Hematocrit 42%
WBCs 7500/mm^3
Platelets 200,000/mm^3

The metabolic profile shows:

Glucose 144 mg/dL
Sodium 133 mEq/L
Potassium 4.1 mEq/L
Chloride 102 mEq/L
BUN 13 mg/dL
Creatinine 0.7 mg/dL.
Blood alcohol level 0.14%

Arterial blood gases:

pH 7.30
Paco$_2$ 56 mm Hg
HCO$_3$ 22 MEq/L
Pao$_2$ 65 mm Hg
O$_2$ saturation 88%

8. Based on the laboratory values, which collaborative intervention will you anticipate next?
   1. Type and cross-match for 3 units of packed red blood cells.
   2. Increase rate of lactated Ringer's solution to 200 mL/hour.
   3. Give lispro insulin using the hospital's standard sliding scale.
   4. Obtain endotracheal intubation tray and assist with intubation.

9. The ED physician writes these additional orders. Which one will you implement first?
   1. Administer metoclopramide (Reglan) 10 mg IV.
   2. Obtain head, chest, and abdomen CT scan, spine and leg x-rays.
   3. Clean occipital laceration and apply antibiotic ointment.
   4. Administer cefuroxime (Zinacef) 1.5 g IV.

The CT scan and x-rays reveal that Ms. A. has a large left frontoparietal lobe epidural hematoma. In addition, she has a left femur fracture and evidence of aspiration pneumonia.

When you reassess Ms. A. after the CT scan, she is flaccid, with no response to verbal or painful stimulation. Her pupils are dilated and non-reactive to light. Her vital signs are:

Blood pressure	190/40 mm Hg
Pulse	40 (sinus bradycardia)
Respirations	14 (ventilator-controlled)
Temperature	96.0°F (axillary)
O$_2$ saturation	92%

10. Which complication are you most concerned about at present?
    1. Brain stem herniation
    2. Respiratory acidosis
    3. Hemorrhage
    4. Hypothermia

Ms. A. is transported to the operating room, where the epidural hematoma is evacuated and an open reduction and internal fixation (ORIF) of her left leg fracture is completed.

After surgery, Ms. A. is transferred to the ICU. She is on a cardiac monitor and has an arterial line in place in her left radial artery. She is making no spontaneous respiratory effort, but is being mechanically ventilated with a ventilator in the assist/control mode at a rate of 14. Ms. A. has a retention catheter, which is draining large amounts of clear, pale yellow urine. An intracranial monitor is in place. Her vital signs are:

Blood pressure	105/54 mm Hg (mean arterial pressure [MAP] 71 mm Hg)
Pulse	50–56 (sinus bradycardia)
Respirations	14 (ventilator controlled)
Temperature	97.4°F (axillary)
O$_2$ saturation	93%
Intracranial pressure (ICP)	17 mm Hg

11. Which of the assessment data listed above requires the most immediate nursing action?
    1. Cardiac rhythm
    2. Blood pressure
    3. Oxygen saturation
    4. Intracranial pressure

12. All of these collaborative and nursing interventions are included in the post-craniotomy plan of care. Which ones are used to meet the goal of maintaining Ms. A.'s cerebral perfusion pressure (CPP) at 70 mm Hg or more? (Choose all that apply.)
    1. Administer dexamethasone (Decadron) 4 mg IV every 8 hours.
    2. Keep head of bed elevated 30 degrees.
    3. Check pupil reaction to light every hour.
    4. Reposition client at least every 2 hours.
    5. Perform endotracheal suctioning as necessary.
    6. Monitor Glasgow Coma Scale hourly.
    7. Administer mannitol (Osmitrol) 100 mg IV PRN if ICP >20 mm Hg.

When you assess Ms. A. on the first post-operative day, her neurologic status has improved a little. She still does not open her eyes to verbal or painful stimuli or respond to commands. She flexes her arms and extends her legs when you apply nailbed pressure. You are unable to assess her verbal response because she is intubated and receiving mechanical ventilation. The right pupil is still larger than the left, but both pupils do react to light. Her GCS is 5. Vital signs are:

Blood pressure	138/85 mm Hg (MAP 99 mm Hg)
Pulse	56 (sinus bradycardia)
Respirations	24 (ventilator-controlled)
Temperature	101.1°F (axillary)
O_2 saturation	99%
ICP	12 mm Hg

13. The post-craniotomy care plan for the first post-operative day includes all of these nursing actions. Which are best delegated to an experienced LPN/LVN working with you in ICU? (Choose all that apply.)
    1. Check gastric pH every 4 hours.
    2. Perform neurologic status examination every 2 hours.
    3. Assess breath sounds every 4 hours.
    4. Check endotracheal tube cuff pressure each shift.
    5. Turn client side to side every 2 hours.
    6. Monitor intake and output hourly.
    7. Send urine specimen for specific gravity daily.
    8. Administer acetaminophen (Tylenol) elixir 625 mg per OG tube PRN if temperature > 101°F.

Arterial blood gases at 7:00 AM on the first post-operative day are:

pH	7.54
$Paco_2$	25 mm Hg
HCO_3	20 mEq/L
Pao_2	110 mm Hg
O_2 saturation	100%

14. Which of these values indicates a need for an immediate change in the ventilator settings?
    1. Pa_{CO_2}
    2. O_2 saturation
    3. HCO_3
    4. Pa_{O_2}

15. At 10:00, the LPN/LVN tells you that Ms. A.'s output for the last hour was 1200 mL and that her urine is very pale yellow. Which action is best to take next?
    1. Instruct the LPN/LVN to continue to monitor the urine output hourly.
    2. Have the LPN/LVN send a urine specimen for specific gravity to the laboratory.
    3. Notify the physician and obtain an order to increase the IV rate.
    4. Assess the neurologic status for signs of increased irritability.

16. Ms. A.'s mother, who has been staying at the bedside, asks you why her daughter is receiving famotidine (Pepcid) since she has no history of peptic ulcers. Which of these answers is best?
    1. Famotidine will lower the chance that she will aspirate.
    2. Famotidine decreases the incidence of gastric stress ulcers.
    3. Famotidine will reduce the risk for gastroesophageal reflux.
    4. Famotidine prevents gastric irritation caused by the orogastric tube.

17. About 20 minutes after you assist the LPN/LVN in repositioning Ms. A. onto her right side, you notice that her ICP has increased to 30 mm Hg. Ms. A.'s BP is 120/55 (MAP − 77). The cardiac monitor shows sinus bradycardia, rate 42. Which is the most appropriate nursing action to accomplish next?
    1. Administer the PRN mannitol 100 mg IV.
    2. Assess the alignment of Ms. A.'s head and neck.
    3. Elevate the head of the bed to 45 degrees.
    4. Check Ms. A.'s pupil size and response to light.

18. When you assess Ms. A. at 2:00 PM, there is little change in her neurologic status. Her left leg, however, is pale, swollen, and very firm when you palpate it. The left leg pulses are only faintly audible using a Doppler. Which action is most appropriate at this time?
    1. Call the orthopedic surgeon to communicate your assessment.
    2. Elevate the left leg on two pillows to decrease the swelling.
    3. Continue to monitor the left leg appearance and pedal pulses.
    4. Assess the client for indications of pain such as restlessness.

19. As your shift ends, you are preparing Ms. A. to transfer to surgery for an emergency fasciotomy. What is your best choice for obtaining informed consent for the fasciotomy?
    1. Informed consent is not needed for emergency surgery.
    2. Permission for surgery can be given by Ms. A.'s mother.
    3. Consent for surgery is not required for unconscious clients.
    4. Authorization can be given by the nursing supervisor.

Mitral Valve Disease and Shortness of Breath

You are assigned to care for Ms. C., an 81-year-old client in the coronary care unit (CCU) who was admitted today with symptoms of increasing shortness of breath over the last week. You are familiar with Ms. C., who has a history of mitral valve regurgitation with left ventricular enlargement and has been admitted multiple times to the CCU and coronary step-down unit. The RN who admitted Ms. C. tells you that she received furosemide (Lasix) 100 mg IV in the emergency department (ED) and her dyspnea has improved. She is receiving oxygen using a nasal cannula at 3 L/minute. She has crackles in both lung bases and her cardiac monitor shows a sinus rhythm, rate 94–96, with occasional premature ventricular contractions (PVCs). The only medication currently ordered is morphine sulfate 2–4 mg IV as needed for chest pain or dyspnea.

Unfortunately, Ms. C.'s condition has deteriorated when you go into the room to assess her. You find that she is sitting up in bed at a 60-degree angle. She is pale, with circumoral cyanosis, and her respirations appear labored and rapid. You ask if she feels more short of breath. Because she is unable to catch her breath enough to speak, she nods her head "yes."

1. What action should you take first?
   1. Listen to her breath sounds.
   2. Ask when the dyspnea started.
   3. Increase her oxygen flow rate to 6 L/minute.
   4. Raise the head of the bed to 75–85 degrees.

When you assess her, you find that she has crackles audible throughout both lung fields and is coughing up pink, frothy sputum. Her oxygen saturation is 85% with the oxygen turned up to 6 L/minute. Her respiratory rate is 38 breaths/minute. She also has 3–4+ pitting edema in her feet and to mid-calf. Even though you have the bed elevated to a 75-degree angle, you can see her jugular veins distended up to her jawline.

2. Which one of these complications are you most concerned about, based on your assessment?
   1. Pulmonary edema
   2. Cor pulmonale
   3. Myocardial infarction
   4. Pulmonary embolus

3. Which action will you take next?
   1. Call the physician about the client's condition.
   2. Place the client on a non-rebreather mask with F_{IO_2} at 95%.
   3. Assist the client to cough and deep breathe.
   4. Administer the ordered morphine sulfate 2 mg IV to the client

4. What additional assessment data are most important to obtain at this time?
   1. Skin color and capillary refill
   2. Orientation and pupil reaction to light
   3. Heart sounds and point of maximum impulse
   4. Blood pressure (BP) and apical pulse

5. Ms. C.'s BP is 98/52 and her apical pulse is 116 and irregular. The cardiac monitor shows sinus tachycardia, rate 110–120, with frequent multifocal PVCs. You call Ms. C.'s physician and receive these orders. Which one will you implement first?
   1. Obtain serum digoxin level.
   2. Give furosemide (Lasix) 100 mg IV.
   3. Check blood potassium level.
   4. Insert #16 French Foley catheter.

6. Which of the orders listed in question 5 is best to delegate to the experienced LPN/LVN who is assisting you?

---

7. While you are waiting for the potassium level to be processed, you administer morphine sulfate 2 mg to Ms. C. A new graduate RN who has just started in CCU asks why you are giving the morphine. What is the best response?
   1. "The morphine will help prevent any chest discomfort from occurring."
   2. "The morphine will decrease Ms. C.'s respiratory rate."
   3. "The morphine will make Ms. C. more comfortable if she has to be intubated."
   4. "The morphine will decrease venous return to the heart."

8. Ms. C.'s potassium level, faxed to the CCU, is 3.1 mEq/L. You call the physician and receive orders to administer potassium chloride (KCl) 20 mEq IV before administering the furosemide. How will you administer the KCl?
   1. Utilize a syringe pump to infuse the KCl over 10 minutes.
   2. Dilute the KCl in 100 mL of D_5W and infuse over 1 hour.
   3. Use a 5-mL syringe and push the KCl over at least 1 minute.
   4. Add the KCl to 1 liter of D_5W and administer over 8 hours.

9. After you have infused the KCl, you administer the furosemide to Ms. C. Which of these nursing actions will be most useful in evaluating whether the furosemide is having the desired effect?
   1. Obtain the client's daily weight.
   2. Measure the hourly urine output.
   3. Monitor blood pressure.
   4. Assess the lung sounds.

10. Ms. C.'s physician arrives and, after assessing her status, leaves an order for nesiritide (Natrecor) 100 mcg (2 mcg/kg) IV bolus, followed by a continuous IV infusion of 0.5 mcg/minute (0.01 mcg/kg/minute). Which client assessment is most important to monitor during the nesiritide infusion?
    1. Lung sounds
    2. Heart rate
    3. Blood pressure
    4. Peripheral edema

11. You are preparing to leave at the end of your shift. Which of these nurses is the best to assign to care for Ms. C.?
    1. A float RN who has worked on the coronary step-down unit for 9 years and has floated before to CCU
    2. An RN from a staffing agency who has 5 years of CCU experience and is orienting to your CCU today
    3. A CCU RN who is already assigned to care for a newly admitted client with chest trauma
    4. The new graduate RN who needs more experience in caring for clients with left ventricular failure

When you return a few days later, Ms. C. has improved enough to transfer to the coronary step-down unit. Her weight has decreased 4 kg from the admission weight. She denies shortness of breath at rest and she has crackles only at the lung bases. She is receiving oxygen at 1 L/minute per nasal cannula. When taking her apical pulse, you notice that she does have a grade III/IV murmur at the apex of the heart and that her pulse is very irregular. The cardiac monitor shows atrial fibrillation, rate 80–100. Ms. C. denies dizziness, but says that her vision feels "fuzzy." She has 2+ pitting ankle edema. Her vital signs are:

Blood pressure	108/62
Pulse	86
Respiratory rate	24
Temperature	97.8°F
O_2 saturation	95%

Her medications are:

> furosemide (Lasix) 40 mg PO twice daily
> aspirin (Ecotrin) 81 mg PO daily
> potassium chloride (K-Dur) 10 mEq daily
> captopril (Capoten) 6.25 mg PO three times daily
> digoxin (Lanoxin) 0.25 mg PO daily

12. Which information in your assessment is most important to report to the physician?
    1. Crackles and oxygen saturation
    2. Atrial fibrillation and fuzzy vision
    3. Apical murmur and pulse rate
    4. Peripheral edema and weight

13. All of Ms. C.'s ordered medications are scheduled for 9:00 AM. Which ones will you hold until you have discussed them with her physician?

Ms. C. is discharged 2 days later. Her discharge medications are:

> furosemide (Lasix) 40 mg PO twice daily
> aspirin (Ecotrin) 81 mg PO daily
> potassium chloride (K-Dur) 10 mEq three times daily
> captopril (Capoten) 6.25 mg PO three times daily
> digoxin (Lanoxin) 0.125 mg PO every other day

In addition, the physician orders a new medication, carvedilol (Coreg) 3.125 mg PO twice daily, and home health visits for Ms. C.

14. Which information will you include when completing Ms. C.'s discharge teaching? (Choose all that apply.)
    1. Weigh yourself first thing in the morning.
    2. Call the doctor if your weight increases more than 5 pounds in 1 day.
    3. Call the doctor if you feel more short of breath or get tired more easily.
    4. Do not take the digoxin if your radial pulse is less than 60.
    5. Take the furosemide first thing in the morning and again at bedtime.
    6. Drink at least 2500 mL of fluids daily.
    7. Move slowly when changing from a lying to a standing position.

When Ms. C. is visited by the home health nurse the next week, she tells the nurse that she feels "more tired now than when I left the hospital." In addition, she is concerned because she's noticed her ankles swelling during the day and "even though I am on a much lower dose of digoxin than I used to be, my pulse rate has been 54 to 58." She has called the doctor's office and been told to continue all her medications as ordered.

15. Based on this information, what nursing action is indicated for Ms. C.?
    1. Teach her about the expected effects of carvedilol.
    2. Place her on a 1000 mL/daily fluid restriction.
    3. Transport her to the ED for treatment.
    4. Encourage her to go to bed earlier in the evening.

Multiple Patients with Peripheral Vascular Disease

You are the team leader working with an LPN/LVN, an experienced nursing assistant, and a nursing student to provide nursing care for six patients in a vascular surgery unit. The patients are as follows:

- *Ms. C., a 38-year-old woman with Raynaud's disease who complains of numbness, tingling, and cold in wrists and hands bilaterally*
- *Mr. R., a 57-year-old man with chronic peripheral arterial disease who complains of severe pain due to an arterial ulcer on his left great toe*
- *Mr. Z., a 44-year- old man with Buerger's disease who wants to discuss enrolling in a smoking cessation program*
- *Ms. Q., a 69-year-old woman with chronic hypertension, her blood pressure (BP) at the end of night shift was 208/96*
- *Mr. S., a 72-year-old man with rule out abdominal aortic aneurysm who is complaining of severe, worsening back pain*
- *Ms. A., a 65-year-old woman with peripheral venous disease and calf swelling who is scheduled for Doppler flow studies this morning*

1. After change of shift report, you make rounds. List the priority order for assessing your patients.
   1. Ms. C.
   2. Mr. R.
   3. Mr. Z.
   4. Ms. Q.
   5. Mr. S.
   6. Ms. A.

   ____, ____, ____, ____, ____, ____

2. When assessing Mr. S., which assessment technique would you instruct the student nurse to avoid?
   1. Auscultate the abdomen for a bruit.
   2. Palpate the abdomen to detect a mass.
   3. Observe the abdomen for a pulsation.
   4. Perform a pain assessment.

3. Mr. S. continues to complain of severe back pain. On assessment you detect a bruit and notice pulsation in the left lower quadrant. What is your best first action?
    1. Measure abdominal girth.
    2. Place patient in high sitting position.
    3. Notify the patient's physician.
    4. Administer pain medication.

4. All of the following orders for Mr. S. are placed by the physician. Which action should you delegate to the LPN/LVN?
    1. Insert a Foley catheter.
    2. Give morphine 2 mg IV push.
    3. Place a second IV heparin lock.
    4. Take vital signs every 15 minutes.

5. Computed tomography (CT) scan reveals that Mr. S. has an aneurysm that is 7.5 cm in diameter. Which preoperative care should the nurse delegate to the nursing student under her supervision? (Choose all that apply).
    1. Teach Mr. S. about coughing and deep breathing.
    2. Assess all peripheral pulses for post-operative comparison.
    3. Administer bowel preparation magnesium sulfate orally.
    4. Draw blood for laboratory to type and screen.
    5. Discuss the reasons for the surgery.

6. Mr. S. is now 1 day post-operative. The student nurse reports that the patient has no bowel sounds present. What is your best action?
    1. Check the nasogastric (NG) tube for kinks.
    2. Notify the surgeon immediately.
    3. Obtain an abdominal x-ray STAT.
    4. Document the finding in the chart.

7. At 8:30 AM, the nursing assistant reports that Ms. Q.'s blood pressure is 198/94. What is the best action to delegate?
    1. Have the LPN/LVN give Ms. Q.'s 9 AM furosemide and enalapril now.
    2. Instruct the nursing assistant to get Ms. Q. back into bed immediately.
    3. Tell the nursing assistant to retake Ms. Q.'s blood pressure every 15 minutes.
    4. Send the LPN/LVN to recheck Ms. Q.'s blood pressure to ensure that the reading is correct.

8. Mr. R. has a nursing diagnosis of Chronic Pain. For which action by the student nurse must you intervene?
    1. Nursing student administers narcotic analgesic 45 minutes before ulcer dressing change.
    2. Nursing student asks the patient if he has ever tried progressive muscle relaxation.
    3. Nursing student assesses the patient's response to pain medication administration.
    4. Nursing student agrees to hold the patient's docusate because of patient request.

9. At noon the LPN/LVN goes to cardiopulmonary resuscitation (CPR) training and is replaced by an RN pulled from the post-anesthesia care unit (PACU). Which patient(s) should you assign to the PACU RN?
    1. Ms. C., who needs teaching about how to avoid exacerbation of symptoms for her condition
    2. Mr. Z., who still needs information about available smoking cessation programs
    3. Ms. Q., whose blood pressure is still elevated and needs frequent blood pressure monitoring
    4. Ms. A., who is worried because the doctor just told her she has a deep vein thrombosis (DVT)

10. You are preparing a teaching plan for Ms. C. with Raynaud's disease. Which key points should you include? (Choose all that apply.)
    1. Avoid exposure to cold by wearing warm clothes.
    2. The nifedipine will help decrease and relieve your symptoms.
    3. Keep your home at a comfortably warm temperature.
    4. The problems you experience are due to vasoconstriction.
    5. Stress reduction techniques can help prevent symptoms.

11. Ms. C. with Raynaud's disease has a nursing diagnosis of Peripheral Ineffective Tissue Perfusion. Which action(s) should you delegate to the experienced nursing assistant? (Choose all that apply.)
    1. Assess for peripheral pulses, edema, capillary refill, and skin temperature.
    2. Inspect skin for presence of tissue breakdown and arterial ulcers.
    3. Remind patient to perform active range-of-motion exercises as tolerated.
    4. Reinforce with patient the need to take in adequate fluids during the day.

12. Ms A. asks why she must have an injection of heparin. What is your best response?
    1. "Heparin will dissolve the clots in your legs."
    2. "Heparin will prevent new clots from forming."
    3. "Heparin will thin your blood and slow down clotting."
    4. "Heparin will prevent the clots from migrating to your lungs."

13. Ms. A. has a nursing diagnosis of Risk for Injury. Which action will you delegate to the nursing assistant?
    1. Assist patient with morning care and ambulation to bathroom.
    2. Monitor patient's daily INR and PTT laboratory results.
    3. Check patient every 4 hours for signs of bleeding.
    4. Tell patient to call for assistance when getting out of bed.

14. The nursing assistant reports that Mr. Z. awoke from a nap complaining of pain in the arch of his left foot. Which of the following action(s) should you take? (Choose all that apply.)
    1. Assess the patient's pain.
    2. Initiate consult for smoking cessation.
    3. Place patient in supine position and elevate foot.
    4. Administer oral analgesics.
    5. Instruct patient to avoid cold temperatures.

15. You are reviewing the lipid profile for a patient with atherosclerosis. Which finding is of most concern?
    1. Total serum cholesterol 220 mg/dL.
    2. Triglycerides of 165 mg/dL
    3. Low-density lipoprotein (LDL) cholesterol of 104 mg/dL
    4. High-density lipoprotein (HDL) cholesterol of 25 mg/dL

Respiratory Difficulty After Surgery

You arrive for your shift on the intensive care step-down unit and receive a change-of-shift report from the previous nurse about Mr. E. Mr. E. is a 26-year-old who was admitted 2 days ago with acute abdominal pain and had an emergency appendectomy. Mr. E.'s appendix had ruptured by the time he came to the hospital, so his surgery was lengthy and required multiple irrigations of the peritoneal cavity. He has a Jackson-Pratt drain in place near his abdominal incision that has been draining moderate amounts of brown purulent fluid. He has a few bowel sounds and has been taking sips of water and ice chips without any nausea or abdominal discomfort. His abdominal dressing is dry and intact. Mr. E.'s wife and sister are sitting with him in his room.

Mr. E. is receiving oxygen at 1 L/minute per nasal cannula. His pulse oximetry had been running 95% to 99%, but over the last 4 hours has decreased to 89% to 90%. There is an order to titrate oxygen to keep his oxygen saturation at 90% or greater. His breath sounds have been decreased at the bases, with a few scattered crackles audible bilaterally. He cooperates when asked to cough, but his cough has been non-productive. His indwelling catheter is draining clear yellow urine. The intake for the last 8 hours was 800 mL; his urine output was 625 mL.

Mr. E.'s cardiac monitor shows a sinus tachycardia, rate 102. When his vital signs were obtained an hour ago, his blood pressure was 148/76, pulse 108, respirations 28, and temperature 101.4° F orally.

Mr. E. is receiving gentamicin (Gentacidin) 100 mg IV every 8 hours and ceftriaxone (Rocephin) 1 g IV every 12 hours. He has morphine sulfate 2–4 mg IV ordered for pain control and received 26 mg of morphine over the previous 8 hours. He has an IV of D_5 ½ normal saline infusing through a dual-lumen subclavian catheter at 80 mL/hour.

Arterial blood gases (ABGs) and a complete blood count (CBC) have just been drawn, but have not been faxed to the unit yet. In addition, electrolytes, blood urea nitrogen (BUN), creatinine, and glucose levels were drawn. Gentamicin peak and trough levels are ordered for today, but have not yet been obtained.

1. Based on the information you have been given during change-of-shift report, what is your greatest concern for Mr. E.?
   1. Purulent abdominal drainage
   2. Sinus tachycardia
   3. Decreased oxygen saturation
   4. Elevated temperature

2. You review Mr. E.'s medications and note that he has a dose of gentamicin scheduled at 10 AM. When will you ask the laboratory to draw blood for the gentamicin trough level?
   1. 9:00 AM
   2. 9:45 AM
   3. 11:30 AM
   4. 2:00 PM

When you go into Mr. E.'s room to assess him, you find him sitting in a chair at the bedside. His respiratory effort looks labored, with a rate of 30 breaths/minute. His continuous pulse oximetry indicates that his oxygen saturation is 88% to 89%. He looks a little anxious and says, "I am having a little trouble catching my breath." His lung sounds are still decreased at the bases, with persistent fine crackles.

3. What action will you take next?
   1. Assist him back to bed.
   2. Increase the oxygen flow rate to 6 L/minute.
   3. Administer morphine IV.
   4. Finish the rest of his head-to-toe assessment.

The ABGs are completed and faxed to the unit:

pH	7.34
$Paco_2$	30 mm Hg
Pao_2	54 mm Hg
HCO_3	20 mEq/L
O_2 saturation	88%

4. Which change in therapy do you anticipate based on the ABGs?
   1. Place Mr. E. on a non-rebreather mask at 15 L/minute.
   2. Administer sodium bicarbonate 50 mEq IV.
   3. Administer morphine to slow the respiratory rate.
   4. The ABG results do not support the need for any change.

5. The CBC results are also available. Which of the results are you most concerned about?
   1. Hemoglobin 10.5 g/dL
   2. Hematocrit 37%
   3. White blood cells 24,000/mm³
   4. Platelets 120,000/mm³

You realize that Mr. E.'s condition is unstable and you will not have time to assess or provide care for your other assigned client, Ms. O. Ms. O. is a diabetic who was admitted yesterday with a urinary tract infection and hyperglycemia. She is receiving a regular insulin infusion (using the hospital's standard insulin sliding scale protocols) and needs to have blood glucose monitoring every hour. Her temperature has decreased from 102°F to 100.6°F since IV ceftizoxime (Cefizox) was started yesterday.

6. Which of these staff members is best to assign to care for Ms. O.?
   1. An RN who has 10 years of experience on the pediatric unit and has floated to the step-down unit for the day.
   2. A new graduate RN who has finished a 3-month orientation and is scheduled for the first day without a preceptor.
   3. An on-call RN with 5 years of experience on the step-down unit who will be able to arrive in about 1 hour.
   4. An experienced RN from a staffing agency who is orienting to the unit today in preparation for a 6-month assignment.

7. Fifteen minutes after use of the non-rebreather mask for oxygen administration is implemented, Mr. E.'s pulse oximeter still indicates that the oxygen saturation is 88% to 89%. What complication is most likely based on your ongoing assessments of this client?
    1. Aspiration pneumonia
    2. Pulmonary embolism
    3. Spontaneous tension pneumothorax
    4. Acute respiratory distress syndrome

8. Mr. E.'s surgeon arrives and asks the hospital intensivist to consult. The intensivist gives these orders after assessing Mr. E. Which one will you implement first?
    1. Transport client to the intensive care unit.
    2. Prepare for intubation and ventilation.
    3. Administer nebulized albuterol (Proventil) every 4 hours.
    4. Obtain blood, urine, and abdominal drainage cultures.

9. The intensivist proceeds to intubate Mr. E. After intubation, which of these actions is the most accurate way to confirm correct placement of the endotracheal (ET) tube?
    1. Chest x-ray study
    2. Lung auscultation
    3. CO_2 detector
    4. Oxygen saturation

Mr. E.'s ET tube placement is confirmed and the ET tube is secured. You note that the 23-cm mark on the ET tube is at the level of Mr. E.'s teeth. Mr. E. is connected to a positive pressure ventilator with the following settings:

Tidal volume (V_T)	800 mL
Rate	14
FIO_2	60%
PEEP	10 cm
Mode	SIMV (synchronized intermittent mandatory ventilation)

ABGs are obtained 30 minutes after Mr. E. is placed on the ventilator:

pH	7.31
$Paco_2$	50 mm Hg
Pao_2	60 mm Hg
HCO_3	20
O_2 saturation	90%

10. Which ventilator change do you anticipate based on your analysis of these ABGs?
    1. Increase the FIO_2 to 70%.
    2. Change the rate on the ventilator to 20 breaths/minute.
    3. Increase the V_T to 1000 mL.
    4. Change to continuous mandatory ventilation (CMV) mode.

After Mr. E. is transferred to the intensive care unit (ICU), you assist with the insertion of a pulmonary artery (PA) catheter (Swan-Ganz catheter) so that pulmonary artery wedge pressure (PAWP) can be monitored. An arterial line is also inserted into the left radial artery. In addition, you insert a nasogastric (NG) tube and connect it to low intermittent suction.

When you re-assess Mr. E., he has scattered crackles audible throughout both lung fields. He is restless and needs frequent reminding not to pull on the ET tube or NG tube. His urine output over the last 2 hours has been 50 mL of clear amber urine. His bowel sounds are slightly hypotonic but are audible in all four abdominal quadrants. His abdominal dressing is still dry and intact and the drainage in the Jackson-Pratt drain is unchanged. You obtain these vital signs for Mr. E.:

Blood pressure	100/46
Pulse	124 (sinus tachycardia)
Respirations	24
Temperature	102.1°F
PAWP	3 mm Hg
Oxygen saturation	90%

11. Based on these data, which collaborative interventions will you anticipate for Mr. E.? (Choose all that apply.)
    1. Increase IV rate to 150 mL/hour.
    2. Administer furosemide (Lasix) 40 mg IV.
    3. Start norepinephrine (Levophed) infusion.
    4. Give diltiazem (Cardizem) 5 mg IV.
    5. Infuse total parenteral nutrition at 70 mL/hour.
    6. Run Ensure enteral feeding at 50 mL/hour.
    7. Give vancomycin (Vancocin) 1000 mg IV.

12. Although his oxygen saturation remains at 90%, Mr. E. continues to be restless and needs frequent reminders to not pull at the ET tube. Which of these methods to reduce his anxiety and decrease the risk for accidental extubation will you try first?
    1. Obtain an order to restrain his hands, and apply soft wrist restraints.
    2. Administer neuromuscular blockade medications and sedatives.
    3. Have a family member stay at Mr. E.'s bedside and reassure him.
    4. Remind Mr. E. frequently that he needs the ET tube to breathe.

13. You are working with a student who is preparing to suction Mr. E. Which action by the student requires that you intervene immediately?
    1. The student increases the FIO_2 to 100% for 1 minute before suctioning.
    2. The student uses an open-suction technique to perform the suctioning.
    3. The student administers morphine 2 mg IV prior to starting to suction.
    4. The student applies suction to the catheter while inserting it into the ET tube.

14. All of the following activities are included in the standard plan of care for a client with adult respiratory distress syndrome (ARDS). Which activities can you delegate to an experienced LPN/LVN whom you are working with in the intensive care unit? (Choose all that apply.)
    1. Provide oral care every 2 hours.
    2. Place the client in the prone position for 4 hours every shift.
    3. Check residuals for enteral feedings every 4 hours.
    4. Assess breath sounds every 4 hours.
    5. Check rectal temperature every 4 hours.
    6. Suction endotracheal tube as needed.
    7. Educate the client and family about routine nursing care.
    8. Check PAWP every 2 hours.
    9. Obtain arterial pressures from arterial line every hour.

You are documenting the events of the morning at the ICU nurse's station when you hear the ventilator alarm. You enter the room and find that the high pressure alarm is sounding and that Mr. E. appears very agitated, with a respiratory rate of 40. The continuous pulse oximeter indicates an oxygen saturation of 81%. The blood pressure displayed on the arterial line monitor is 98/44. Mr. E.'s cardiac monitor shows a sinus tachycardia, rate 142.

15. What action will you accomplish first?
    1. Listen to Mr. E.'s breath sounds and assess chest movement.
    2. Use a bag-valve-mask system to manually ventilate Mr. E.
    3. Check the ventilator settings and readouts.
    4. Suction Mr. E. after hyperoxygenating him.

16. You do not hear any breath sounds over Mr. E.'s right side, and the right side does not expand much with inspiration. When you check the location of the ET tube at the client's teeth, you find that it is still at the 23-cm mark. What complication of intubation and mechanical ventilation do you suspect?
    1. Inadvertent extubation
    2. Tension pneumothorax
    3. ET tube displacement
    4. Aspiration pneumonia

17. The intensivist arrives quickly and inserts a chest tube into the right anterior chest at the second intercostal space. You assess Mr. E. after the chest tube insertion. Which of these assessment data is of most concern?
    1. A large number of air bubbles appear in the water seal chamber during expiration.
    2. Continuous bubbling occurs throughout the respiratory cycle in the suction control chamber.
    3. 100 mL of blood drains into the collection chamber immediately after the chest tube insertion.
    4. The client indicates that he has pain with every ventilator-assisted inspiration.

18. Just before you prepare to give a change-of-shift report to the oncoming RN, you review Mr. E.'s other laboratory tests for today. Which of these is most important to communicate to the physician?
    1. Blood glucose 140 mg/dL
    2. Potassium 5.1 mEq/L
    3. Sodium 134 mEq/L
    4. BUN 52 mg/dL

PART 2

Chapter 1: Pain, pages 15—18

1. **Ans: 4**   As charge nurse, you must assess the performance and attitude of the staff in relation to this client. After gathering data from the nurses, additional information from the records and the client can be obtained as necessary. The educator may be of assistance if knowledge deficit or need for performance improvement is the problem. **Focus:** Supervision/prioritization

2. **Ans: 3**   The family is part of the sociocultural dimension of pain. They are influencing the client and should be included in the teaching sessions about the appropriate use of narcotics and about the adverse effects of pain on the healing process. The other dimensions should be included to help the client/family understand the overall treatment plan and pain mechanism. **Focus:** Prioritization

3. **Ans: 1**   Antidepressants such as amitriptyline can be given for diabetic neuropathy. Corticosteroids are for pain associated with inflammation. Methylphenidate is given to counteract sedation if the client is on opioids. Lorazepam is an anxiolytic. **Focus:** Prioritization

4. **Ans: 3**   Cancer pain generally worsens with disease progression and the use of opioids is more generous. Fibromyalgia is more likely to be treated with non-opioid and adjuvant medications. Trigeminal neuralgia is treated with anti-seizure medications such as carbamazepine (Tegretol). Phantom limb pain usually subsides after ambulation begins. **Focus:** Prioritization

5. **Ans: 4**   In supervising the new RN, good performance should be reinforced first and then areas of improvement can be addressed. Asking the nurse about knowledge of pain management is also an option; however, it would be a more indirect and time-consuming approach. Making a note and watching do not help the nurse to correct the immediate problem. In-service might be considered if the problem persists. **Focus:** Supervision/delegation

6. **Ans: 3**   The Faces pain rating scale (depicting smiling, neutral, frowning, crying, etc.) is appropriate for young children who may have difficulty describing pain or understanding the correlation of pain to numerical or verbal descriptors. The other tools require abstract reasoning abilities to make analogies and use of advanced vocabulary. **Focus:** Prioritization

7. **Ans: 3**   The client must be believed and his or her experience of pain must be acknowledged as valid. The data gathered via client reports can then be applied to the other options in developing the treatment plan. **Focus:** Prioritization

8. **Ans: 3**   The IV route is preferred as the fastest and most amenable to titration. A PCA bolus can be delivered; however, the pump will limit the dosage that can be delivered unless the parameters are changed. Intraspinal administration requires special catheter placement and there are more potential complications with this route. Sublingual is reasonably fast, but not a good route for titration, and medication variety in this form is limited. **Focus:** Prioritization

9. **Ans: 1**   The goal is to control pain while minimizing side effects. For severe pain, the medication can be titrated upward until the pain is controlled. Downward titration occurs when the pain begins to subside. Adequate dosing is important; however, the concept of controlled dosing applies more to potent vasoactive drugs. **Focus:** Prioritization

10. **Ans: 2**   Use of heat and cold applications is a standard therapy with guidelines for safe use and predictable outcomes, and an LPN/LVN will be implementing this therapy in the hospital, under the supervision of an RN. Therapeutic touch requires additional training and practice. Meditation is not acceptable to all clients and an assessment of spiritual beliefs should be conducted. Transcutaneous electrical stimulation is usually applied by a physical therapist. **Focus:** Delegation

11. **Ans: 2, 3, 1**   Step 1 includes non-opioids and adjuvant drugs. Step 2 includes opioids for mild pain plus Step 1 drugs and adjuvant drugs as needed. Step 3 includes opioids for severe pain (replacing Step 2 opioids) and continuing Step 1 drugs and adjuvant drugs as needed. **Focus:** Prioritization

12. **Ans: 4**   At greatest risk are elderly clients, opiate naive clients, and those with underlying pulmonary disease. The child has two of the three risk factors. **Focus:** Prioritization

13. **Ans: 1**   This client has strong beliefs and emotions related to the issue of the sibling's addiction. First, encourage expression. This indicates to the client that the feelings are real and valid. It is also an opportunity to assess beliefs and fears. Giving facts and information is appropriate at the right time. Family involvement is important, bearing in mind that their beliefs about drug addiction may be similar to those of the client. **Focus:** Prioritization

14. **Ans: 3**   Diaphoresis is one of the early signs that occur between 6 and 12 hours. Fever, nausea, and abdominal cramps are late signs that occur between 48 and 72 hours. **Focus:** Prioritization

15. **Ans: 1**   The nursing assistant is able to assist the client with hygiene issues and knows the principles of safety and comfort for this procedure. Monitoring the client, teaching techniques, and evaluating outcomes are nursing responsibilities. **Focus:** Delegation

16. **Ans: 4** The charge nurse is a resource person who can help locate and review the policy. If the physician is insistent, he or she could give the placebo personally, but delaying the administration does not endanger the health or safety of the client. While following one's own ethical code is correct, you must ensure that the client is not abandoned and that care continues. **Focus:** Prioritization

17. **Ans: 2** Complete information from the family should be obtained during the initial comprehensive history and assessment. If this information is not obtained, the nursing staff will have to rely on observation of nonverbal behavior and careful documentation to determine pain and relief patterns. **Focus:** Prioritization

18. **Ans: 3** If the gastrointestinal system is functional, the oral route is preferred for routine analgesics because of lower cost and ease of administration. Oral route is also less painful and less invasive than the IV, IM, subcutaneous, or PCA routes. Transdermal route is slower and medication availability is limited compared to oral forms. **Focus:** Prioritization

19. **Ans: 4** Assess the pain for changes in location, quality, and intensity, as well as changes in response to medication. This assessment will guide the next steps. **Focus:** Prioritization

20. **Ans: 3** The side-lying, knee-chest position opens the retroperitoneal space and provides relief. The pillow provides a splinting action. Diversional therapy is not the best choice for acute pain, especially if the activity requires concentration. TENS is more appropriate for chronic muscular pain. The additional stimulation of massage may be distressing for this client. **Focus:** Prioritization

21. **Ans: 4** If the pain is constant, the best schedule is around-the-clock, to provide steady analgesia and pain control. The other options may actually require higher doses to achieve control. **Focus:** Prioritization

22. **Ans: 2, 3** The clients with the cast and the toe amputation are stable clients and need ongoing assessment and pain management that are within the scope of practice for an LPN/LVN under the supervision of an RN. The RN should take responsibility for pre-operative teaching, and the terminal cancer client needs a comprehensive assessment to determine the reason for refusal of medication. **Focus:** Assignment

23. **Ans: 3** When a client takes aspirin, monitor for increases in PT (normal range 11.0–12.5 seconds or 85%–100%). Also monitor for possible decreases in potassium (normal range 3.5–5.0 mEq/L). If bleeding signs are noted, hematocrit should be monitored (normal range male 42%–52%, female 37%–47%). An elevated BUN could be seen if the client is having chronic gastrointestinal bleeding (normal range 10–20 mg/dL). **Focus:** Prioritization

24. **Ans: 2** A second day post-operative client who needs medication prior to dressing changes has predictable and routine care that a new nurse can manage. Although chronic pain clients can be relatively stable, the interaction with this client will be time consuming and may cause the new nurse to fall behind. The HIV client has complex complaints that require expert assessment skills. The client pending discharge will need special and detailed instructions. **Focus:** Assignment

25. **Ans: 3** Directly ask the client about the pain and do a complete pain assessment. This information will determine which action to take next. **Focus:** Prioritization

Chapter 2: Cancer, pages 19–22

1. **Ans: 1** Oral hygiene is within the scope of responsibilities of the nursing assistant. It is the responsibility of the nurse to observe response to treatments and to help the patient deal with loss or anxiety. The nursing assistant can be directed to weigh the patient, but should not be expected to know when to initiate that measurement. **Focus:** Delegation

2. **Ans: 4** The patient's physical condition is currently stable, but emotional needs are affecting his or her ability to receive the information required to make an informed decision. The other diagnoses are relevant, but if the patient leaves the clinic the interventions may be delayed or ignored. **Focus:** Prioritization

3. **Ans: 1** Pancreatic cancer is more common in blacks, males, and smokers. Other links include use of alcohol, diabetes, obesity, history of pancreatitis, organic chemicals, a high-fat diet, and previous abdominal radiation. **Focus:** Prioritization

4. **Ans: 3, 4, 2, 5, 1** This classification system is based on the extent of the disease rather than the histological changes. Stage 0: cancer in situ, stage I: tumor limited to tissue of origin, stage II: limited local spread, stage III: extensive local and regional spread, stage IV: metastasis. **Focus:** Prioritization

5. **Ans: 2** Administering enemas and antibiotics is within the scope of practice for LPN/LVNs. Although some states may allow the LPN/LVN to administer blood, in general, blood administration, pre-operative teaching, and assisting with central line insertion are the responsibilities of the RN. **Focus:** Prioritization

6. **Ans: 1. Nurse practitioner, 2. Nutritionist, 3. LPN/LVN, 4. Nurse practitioner, 5. RN** The nurse practitioner is often the provider who performs the physical examinations and recommends diagnostic testing. The nutritionist can give information about diet. The LPN/LVN will know the standard seven warning signs and can educate through standard teaching programs in some states. However, the RN has primary responsibility for educating people about risk factors. **Focus:** Assignment

7. **Ans: 2** The physician has described a treatment for controlling cancer that is not curable. When the goal is cure, the patient will be deemed free of disease after treatments. In palliation, the treatment is given primarily for pain relief. *Permanent remission* is another term to describe cure. **Focus:** Prioritization

8. **Ans: 3** The nursing assistant can observe the amount that the patient eats (or what is gone from the tray) and report to the nurse. Assessing patterns of fatigue or skin reaction is the responsibility of the RN. The initial recommendation for exercise should come from the physician. **Focus:** Delegation

9. **Ans: 3** Paresthesia is a side effect associated with some chemotherapy drugs such as vincristine (Oncovin). The physician can modify the dose or discontinue the drug. Fatigue, nausea, vomiting, and anorexia are common side effects for many chemotherapy medications. The nurse can assist the patient by planning for rest periods, giving antiemetics as ordered, and encouraging small meals with high-protein and high-calorie foods. **Focus:** Prioritization

10. **Ans: 1** WBC count is especially important because chemotherapy can cause decreases in WBCs, particularly neutrophils, which leaves the patient vulnerable to infection. The other tests are important in the total

management, but less directly specific to chemotherapy. **Focus:** Prioritization

11. **Ans: 3**   Giving medications is within the scope of practice for the LPN/LVN. Assisting the patient to brush and floss should be delegated to the nursing assistant. Explaining contraindications is the responsibility of the RN. Recommendations for saliva substitutes should come from the physician or pharmacist. **Focus:** Delegation

12. **Ans: 1**   Ideally, chemotherapy drugs should be given by nurses who have received additional training in how to safely prepare and deliver the drugs and protect themselves from exposure. The other options are a concern but the general principles of drug administration apply. **Focus:** Assignment

13. **Ans: 1, 3, 2, 4**   Tumor lysis syndrome is an emergency of electrolyte imbalances and potential renal failure. A patient scheduled for surgery should be assessed and prepared for surgery. A patient with breakthrough pain needs assessment and the physician may need to be contacted for a change of dose or medication. Anticipatory nausea and vomiting has a psychogenic component that requires assessment, teaching, reassurance, and antiemetics. **Focus:** Prioritization

14. **Ans: 1**   Back pain is an early sign occurring in 95% of patients. The other symptoms are later signs. **Focus:** Prioritization

15. **Ans: 2, 3, 4, 1**   Induction is the initial aggressive treatment to destroy leukemia cells. Intensification starts immediately after induction, lasting for several months and targeting persistent, undetected leukemia cells. Consolidation occurs after remission to eliminate any remaining leukemia cells. Maintenance involves lower doses to keep the body free of leukemia cells. **Focus:** Prioritization

16. **Ans: 4**   T (tumor) 0–4 signifies tumors of increasing size. N (regional lymph nodes) 0–3 signifies increasing involvement of lymph nodes. M (metastasis) 0 signifies no metastasis and 1 signifies distal metastasis. **Focus:** Prioritization

17. **Ans: 2**   Potentially life-threatening hypercalcemia can occur in cancers with destruction of bone. Other laboratory values are pertinent for overall patient management but are less specific to bone cancers. **Focus:** Prioritization

18. **Ans: 2, 4**   Debulking of tumor and laminectomy are palliative procedures. These patients can be placed in the same room. The patient with low neutrophil count and the patient who has had a bone marrow harvest need protective isolation. **Focus:** Assignment

19. **Ans: 1**   Cigarette smoking is associated with 80–90% of lung cancers. Occupational exposure coupled with cigarette smoking increases risks. ETS increases risks by 35%. Cigar smoking provides higher risk than pipe smoking, but both are lower risks than cigarette smoking. **Focus:** Prioritization

20. **Ans: 2**   Tumor lysis syndrome can result in severe electrolyte imbalances and potential renal failure. The other laboratory values are important to monitor for general chemotherapy side effects, but are less pertinent to tumor lysis syndrome. **Focus:** Prioritization

21. **Ans: 1, 3**   After age 18, females should have annual Pap smears, regardless of sexual activity. African-American males should begin prostate-specific antigen testing at age 45. Annual mammograms are recommended for women over the age of 40. Annual fecal occult blood

testing is recommended starting at age 50. **Focus:** Prioritization

22. **Ans: 2**   Hyponatremia is a concern; therefore, fluid restrictions would be ordered. Urinalysis is less pertinent; however, the nurse should monitor for increased urine specific gravity. The diet may need to include sodium supplements. Fluid bolus is unlikely to be ordered for SIADH. **Focus:** Prioritization

23. **Ans: 1, 2, 4, 6**   Vital signs and reporting on specific parameters, good handwashing, and gathering equipment are within the scope of duties for a nursing assistant. Assessing for symptoms of infection/superinfections is the responsibility of the RN. **Focus:** Delegation

24. **Ans: 2**   The LPN/LVN is versed in medication administration and able to teach patients standardized information. The other options require more in-depth assessment, planning, and teaching, which should be performed by the RN. **Focus:** Delegation

Chapter 3: Fluid, Electrolyte, and Acid-Base Problems, pages 23–26

1. **Ans: 2**   The nursing assistant can reinforce additional fluid intake once it is part of the care plan. Administering IV fluids, developing plans, and teaching families require additional education and skills that are within the scope of practice for the RN. **Focus:** Delegation/supervision

2. **Ans: 1**   Normally, neck veins are distended when the client is in the supine position. These veins flatten as the client moves to a sitting position. The other three responses are characteristic of Excess Fluid Volume. **Focus:** Prioritization

3. **Ans: 1, 2, 3, 4**   The LPN/LVN's scope of practice and educational preparation includes oral care and routine observation. State practice acts vary as to whether LPN/LVNs are permitted to perform assessment. The client should be reminded to avoid most commercial mouthwashes that contain alcohol, a drying agent. Initiating a dietary consult is within the purview of the RN or physician. **Focus:** Delegation/supervision

4. **Ans: 4**   Bilateral moist crackles indicate fluid-filled alveoli, which interferes with gas exchange. Furosemide is a potent loop diuretic that will help mobilize the fluid in the lungs. The other orders are important but not urgent. **Focus:** Prioritization

5. **Ans: 2**   Suspect hypokalemia and check the client's potassium level. Common ECG changes with hypokalemia include ST depression, inverted T waves, and prominent U waves. Clients with hypokalemia may also develop heart block. **Focus:** Prioritization

6. **Ans: 1**   The client's potassium is high (normal range 3.5–5.0). Kayexalate removes potassium from the body through the gastrointestinal system. Spironolactone is a potassium-sparing diuretic that may cause the client's potassium level to go even higher. The nursing student may not have the skill to assess ECG strips and this should be done by the RN. **Focus:** Delegation/supervision

7. **Ans: 3**   SIADH causes a relative sodium deficit due to excessive retention of water. **Focus:** Prioritization

8. **Ans: 1**   Providing oral care is within the scope of practice for the nursing assistant. Monitoring and assessing clients, as well as administering IV fluids, require the additional education and skills of the RN. **Focus:** Assignment, delegation/supervision

9. **Ans: 2** A positive Chvostek's sign (facial twitching of one side of the mouth, nose, and cheek in response to tapping the face just below and in front of the ear) is a neurologic manifestation of hypocalcemia. The LPN/LVN is experienced and possesses the skills to take accurate vital signs. **Focus:** Prioritization

10. **Ans: 4** Clients with low calcium levels should be encouraged to consume dairy products, seafood, nuts, broccoli, and spinach, which are all good sources of dietary calcium. **Focus:** Prioritization

11. **Ans: 3** A musculoskeletal manifestation of low phosphorus is generalized muscle weakness that may lead to acute muscle breakdown (rhabdomyolysis). Even though the other statements are true, they do not answer the nursing assistant's question. **Focus:** Delegation/supervision

12. **Ans: 4** While all of these laboratory values are outside of the normal range, the magnesium is most outside of normal. With a magnesium level this low, the client is at risk for ECG changes and life-threatening ventricular dysrhythmias. **Focus:** Prioritization

13. **Ans: 2** The client with COPD, although ventilator dependent, is the most stable of this group. Clients with acid-base imbalances often require frequent laboratory assessment and changes in therapy to correct their disorders. In addition, the client with DKA is a new admission and will require an in-depth admission assessment. All three of these clients need care from an experienced critical care nurse. **Focus:** Assignment

14. **Ans: 1** The blood gas component responsible for respiratory acidosis is CO_2 (carbon dioxide). Increasing the ventilator rate will blow off more CO_2 and decrease the acidosis. Changes in the oxygen setting may improve oxygenation but will not affect respiratory acidosis. **Focus:** Prioritization

15. **Ans: 2, 3** The nursing assistant's training and education include how to take vital signs and record intake and output. The need to take vital signs this frequently indicates that the client may be unstable. The nurse should give the nursing assistant reporting parameters when delegating this action, and should also check the vital signs for indications in instability. Performing fingerstick glucose checks and assessing clients require additional education and skill that are appropriate to licensed nurses. Some facilities may train experienced nursing assistants to perform fingerstick glucose checks and change their role descriptions to designate their new skills, but this is beyond the normal scope of practice for a nursing assistant. **Focus:** Delegation/supervision

16. **Ans: 4** Risk factors for acid-base imbalances in the older adult include chronic renal disease and pulmonary disease. Occasional antacid use will not cause imbalances, although antacid abuse is a risk factor for metabolic alkalosis. **Focus:** Prioritization

17. **Ans: 1** A decreased respiratory rate indicates respiratory depression which also puts the client at risk for respiratory acidosis. All of the other findings are important and should be reported to the RN, but the respiratory rate is urgent. **Focus:** Delegation/supervision

18. **Ans: 2** The client is most likely hyperventilating and blowing off CO_2. This decrease in CO_2 will lead to an increase in pH, causing a respiratory alkalosis. Respiratory acidosis results from respiratory depression and retained CO_2. Metabolic acidosis and alkalosis result from problems related to renal acid-base control. **Focus:** Prioritization, supervision

19. **Ans: 1** Prolonged nausea and vomiting can result in acid deficit that can lead to metabolic alkalosis. The other findings are important and need to be assessed but are not related to acid-base imbalances. **Focus:** Prioritization, supervision

20. **Ans: 2** Nasogastric suctioning can result in a decrease in acid components and a metabolic alkalosis. The client's increase in rate and depth of ventilation is an attempt to compensate by blowing off CO_2. The first response may be true but does not address all the components of the question. The third and fourth answers are inaccurate. **Focus:** Supervision, prioritization

Chapter 4: Immunologic Problems, pages 27–30

1. **Ans: 3** Epinephrine given rapidly at the onset of an anaphylactic reaction may prevent or reverse cardiovascular collapse as well as airway narrowing caused by bronchospasm and inflammation. Oxygen use is also appropriate, but generally is administered using a non-rebreather mask at 90%–100% FIO_2. Albuterol may also be used to decrease airway narrowing, but would not be the first therapy used for anaphylaxis. An IV access will take longer to establish and should not be the first intervention. **Focus:** Prioritization

2. **Ans: 1** Supplying bleach solution to patients who are at risk for HIV infection can be done by staff members with health assistant education. Pre-operative/post-operative test counseling may be done by non-RN personnel with specialized training; however, an RN would be better prepared to answer questions that are likely to be asked by at-risk individuals. Education and community assessment are RN-level skills. **Focus:** Delegation

3. **Ans: 2** Nystatin should be in contact with the oral and esophageal tissues as long as possible for maximum effect. The other actions are also inappropriate and should be discussed with the student but do not require action as quickly. HIV-positive patients do not require droplet/contact precautions or visitor restrictions for opportunistic infections. Hot or spicy foods are not usually well tolerated by patients with oral or esophageal fungal infections. **Focus:** Prioritization

4. **Ans: 4** Pentamidine can cause fatal hypoglycemia, so the low blood glucose level indicates a need for a change in therapy. The low blood pressure suggests that the IV infusion rate may need to be slowed. The other responses indicate need for independent nursing actions (such as obtaining a new IV site and encouraging oral intake) but are not associated with pentamidine infusion. **Focus:** Prioritization

5. **Ans: 2** Drug therapy for HIV infection requires taking multiple medications on a very consistent schedule. Failure to take the medications consistently can lead to mutations and the emergence of more virulent forms of the virus. Although the other data indicate the need for further assessments or interventions, they will not affect the decision to initiate antiretroviral therapy for this patient. **Focus:** Prioritization

6. **Ans: 3** The staff member who is most knowledgeable about the regulations regarding HIV prophylaxis and obtaining a patient's HIV status and/or patient HIV testing is the occupational health nurse. Doing unauthorized HIV testing or asking the patient yourself would be unethical. The nurse manager is not responsible for obtaining this information (unless the manager

is also in charge of occupational health). **Focus:** Prioritization

7. **Ans: 1** Patients with severe immunodeficiency may be unable to produce an immune response, so a negative TB skin test does not completely rule out a TB diagnosis for this patient. The next steps in diagnosis are a chest x-ray and sputum culture. Teaching about INH and follow-up TB testing may be required, depending on the x-ray and sputum culture results. **Focus:** Prioritization

8. **Ans: 2** Collecting data used to evaluate the therapeutic and adverse effects of medications is included in LPN/LVN education and scope of practice. Assessment, planning, and teaching are more complex skills that will require RN education. Assistance with hygiene and activities of daily living should be delegated to the nursing assistants. **Focus:** Delegation

9. **Ans: 3** To be most effective, cyclosporine must be mixed and administered following the manufacturer's instructions, so the RN who is likely to have the most experience with the medication should care for this patient or monitor the new graduate carefully during medication preparation and administration. The coronary care unit (CCU) float nurse and new orientee would not have experience with this medication. **Focus:** Assignment

10. **Ans: 4** Both naproxen (an NSAID) and prednisone (a corticosteroid) can cause gastrointestinal bleeding and the stool appearance indicates that there may be blood present in the stool. A stool specimen should be checked for occult blood. Also, it is likely that the patient needs to start taking a proton-pump inhibitor such as pantoprazole (Protonix) to reduce gastric acid secretion. The other symptoms are common in patients with RA and will require assessments and interventions, but do not indicate that therapy needs to be altered. **Focus:** Prioritization

11. **Ans: 1** Nausea and vomiting are common adverse effects of interferon alfa-2a, but continued vomiting should be reported to the physician because dehydration may occur. The medication may be given by either the subcutaneous or intramuscular route. Flu-like symptoms such as a mild temperature elevation, headache, muscle aches, and anorexia are common after initiating therapy but tend to decrease over time. **Focus:** Prioritization

12. **Ans: 3** Patients taking immunosuppressive medications are at increased risk for development of cancer. A non-tender swelling or lump may indicate that the patient has lymphoma. The other data indicate that the patient is experiencing common side effects of the immunosuppressive medications. **Focus:** Prioritization

13. **Ans: 1** Taking antiretroviral medications such as indinavir on a rigid time schedule is essential for effective treatment of HIV infection and to avoid development of drug-resistant strains of the virus. The other medications should also be given within the time frame indicated in the hospital policy (usually within 30 minutes of the scheduled time). **Focus:** Prioritization

14. **Ans: 4** Viral load testing measures the amount of HIV genetic material in the blood, so a decrease in viral load indicates that the ART is effective. The lymphocyte count is used to assess the impact of HIV on immune function but will not directly measure the effectiveness of antiretroviral therapy. The ELISA and Western blot tests monitor for the presence of antibodies to HIV, so

these will be positive after the patient is infected with HIV even if drug therapy is effective. **Focus:** Prioritization

15. **Ans: 1** Administration of oral medication is appropriate for LPN education and scope of practice. Oral care should be delegated to a nursing assistant. Teaching and assessment are more complex RN-level interventions. **Focus:** Delegation

16. **Ans: 2** Methotrexate is teratogenic and should not be used in patients who are pregnant. The physician will need to discuss use of contraception during the time the patient is taking methotrexate. The other patient information may require further patient assessment or teaching but does not indicate that methotrexate may be contraindicated for the patient. **Focus:** Prioritizaton

17. **Ans: 2** The varicella (chickenpox) vaccine is a live-virus vaccine and should not be administered to patients who are receiving immunosuppressive medications such as prednisone. The other medical orders are appropriate. Prednisone dose should be tapered gradually when patients have been on long-term steroid therapy, but tapering is not necessary for short-term prednisone use. CRP levels are not the most specific test for monitoring treatment but are inexpensive and frequently used. High doses of NSAIDs such as ibuprofen are more likely to cause side effects such as gastrointestinal bleeding but are useful in treating the joint pain associated with SLE exacerbations. **Focus:** Prioritization

18. **Ans: 3** Albuterol is the most rapid acting of the medications listed. Corticosteroids are helpful in prevention of allergic reactions, but are not as rapid acting. Cromolyn is used as a prophylactic medication to prevent asthma attacks, but not to treat acute attacks. Aminophylline is not a first-line treatment for bronchospasm. **Focus:** Prioritization

19. **Ans: 1** A high number of patients with SLE develop nephropathy, so an increase in BUN may indicate a need for a change in therapy or for further diagnostic testing such as a creatinine clearance test or renal biopsy. The other laboratory results are not unusual in patients with SLE. **Focus:** Prioritization

20. **Ans: 2** Individuals with allergic reactions to these fruits have a high incidence of latex allergy. More information and/or testing is needed to determine whether the new employee has a latex allergy, which might affect ability to provide direct patient care. The other findings would be important to include in documenting the employee's health history, but would not affect ability to provide patient care. **Focus:** Prioritization

Chapter 5: Respiratory Problems, pages 31–36

1. **Ans: 1, 2, 4** The experienced LPN/LVN is capable of gathering data and observations including breath sounds and pulse oximetry. Administering medications, such as MDIs, is within the scope of practice for the LPN/LVN. Independently completing the admission assessment, initiating the nursing care plan, and evaluating a client's abilities require additional education and skills. These actions are within the scope of practice for the professional RN. **Focus:** Delegation/supervision

2. **Ans: 2** For clients with chronic emphysema, the stimulus to breathe is a low serum oxygen level (normal

stimulus is high carbon dioxide level). This client's oxygen flow is too high and is causing a high oxygen level, resulting in a decreased respiratory rate. If you do not intervene, the client is at risk for a respiratory arrest. Crackles, barrel chest, and sitting up leaning over the night-table are common in clients with chronic emphysema. **Focus:** Prioritization

3. **Ans: 1**   When an oxygen flow rate is greater than 4 L/min, the mucous membranes can be dried out. The best treatment is to add humidification to the oxygen delivery system. Application of water-soluble jelly to the nares can also help decrease mucosal irritation. None of the other options will treat the problem. **Focus:** Prioritization

4. **Ans: 3**   When performing tracheostomy care, a sterile field is set up and sterile technique is used. Standard precautions such as washing hands must also be maintained but are not enough when performing tracheostomy care. The presence of a tracheostomy tube provides direct access to the lungs for organisms, so sterile techniques are used to prevent infections. All of the other steps are correct and appropriate. **Focus:** Delegation/supervision

5. **Ans: 2, 3, 4, 5**   The correct position for a client with an anterior nosebleed is upright and leaning forward to prevent blood from entering the stomach and prevent possible aspiration. All of the other instructions are appropriate according to best practice for emergency care of a client with an anterior nosebleed. **Focus:** Delegation/supervision, assignment

6. **Ans: 3**   The nursing assistant can remind clients about actions that have already been taught by the nurse and are part of the client's plan of care. Discussing and teaching require additional education and training. These actions fit the scope of practice for the RN. The RN could delegate administration of the medication to the LPN/LVN. **Focus:** Delegation/supervision

7. **Ans: 1, 2**   The new RN is at an early point in her orientation. The most appropriate clients to assign are stable with usual, routine care. The client with the lobectomy will require the care of an experienced nurse with frequent assessments and monitoring for postoperative complications. The client admitted with newly diagnosed esophageal cancer will also benefit from an experienced nurse's care. This client may have questions and needs a comprehensive admission assessment. As the new nurse advances through her orientation, you will want to work with her providing care for these more complex clients. **Focus:** Assignment, delegation/supervision

8. **Ans: 1, 2, 4, 5**   Bedding should be washed with hot water to destroy dust mites. All of the other points are accurate and appropriate to a teaching plan for a client with a new diagnosis of asthma. **Focus:** Prioritization

9. **Ans: 1, 3, 2, 5, 4, 6**   Before each use, the cap is removed and the inhaler is shaken according to the instructions on the package insert. Next the client should tilt the head back and breathe out completely. As the client begins to breathe in deeply through his mouth, the canister should be pressed down to release one puff (dose) of the medication. The client should continue to breathe in slowly over 3–5 seconds and then hold his breath for at least 10 seconds to allow the medication to reach deep into the lungs. Clients should wait at least 1 minute between puffs from the inhaler. **Focus:** Prioritization

10. **Ans: 1**   Assisting clients with positioning and activities of daily living are within the educational preparation and scope of practice of the nursing assistant. Teaching, instructing, and assessing clients all require additional education and skills and are more appropriate to the scope of practice of licensed nurses. **Focus:** Delegation/supervision

11. **Ans: 1**   Experienced LPN/LVNs can use observation of clients to gather data regarding how well clients perform interventions that have already been taught. Assisting clients with ADLs is more appropriately delegated to the nursing assistant. Planning and consulting require additional education and skills that are appropriate to the RN's scope of practice. **Focus:** Delegation/supervision

12. **Ans: 4**   The client who did not have the pneumonia vaccination or the flu shot is at increased risk for developing pneumonia or influenza. An elevated temperature indicates some form of infection, which may be respiratory in origin. All of the other vital signs are fairly normal. **Focus:** Delegation/supervision

13. **Ans: 2**   The nursing assistant's training includes monitoring and recording intake and output. After the nurse has instructed/taught the client about the importance of adequate nutritional intake for energy, the nursing assistant can remind and encourage the client to take in adequate nutrition. Instructing clients and planning activities require more education and skills that are appropriate to the RN's scope of practice. Monitoring the client's cardiovascular response to activity is a complex process requiring additional education, training, and skill, appropriate to the RN's scope of practice. **Focus:** Delegation/supervision

14. **Ans: 2**   Continuous bubbling indicates an air leak that must be identified. With the physician's order you can apply a padded clamp on the drainage tubing close to the occlusive dressing. If the bubbling stops, the air leak may be at the chest tube insertion, which will require you to notify the physician. If the air bubbling does not stop when you apply the padded clamp, the air leak is between the clamp and the drainage system and you must assess the system carefully to locate the leak. Chest tube drainage of 10–15 mL per hour is acceptable. The chest tube dressing is not changed daily, but may be reinforced. The client's complaints of pain need to be assessed and treated. This is important but is not as urgent as a chest tube leak. **Focus:** Delegation/supervision

15. **Ans: 4**   The client with asthma did not achieve relief from SOB after using the bronchodilator and is at risk for respiratory complications. This client's needs are urgent. The other clients need to be assessed as soon as possible but none of them is urgent. COPD clients with pulse oximetry oxygen saturations greater than 90% are acceptable. **Focus:** Prioritization

16. **Ans: 3**   The nursing assistant can remind the client to perform actions that are already part of the plan of care. Assisting the client into the best position to facilitate coughing requires specialized knowledge and understanding that are beyond the scope of the basic nursing assistant. However, an experienced nursing assistant could assist the client with positioning after the nursing assistant and the client had been taught the proper technique. The nursing assistant would still be under the supervision of the RN. Teaching clients

about adequate fluid intake and techniques that facilitate coughing requires additional education and skill and is within the scope of the RN. **Focus:** Delegation/supervision

17. **Ans: 3** Many surgical clients are taught about coughing, deep breathing, and use of incentive spirometry preoperatively. To care for the client with TB on isolation, the nurse must be fitted for a high-efficiency particulate air (HEPA) respirator mask. The bronchoscopy client needs specialized and careful assessment and monitoring after the procedure, and the ventilator-dependent client needs a nurse who is familiar with ventilator care. Both of these clients need experienced nurses. **Focus:** Assignment

18. **Ans: 2** Clients taking INH must continue the drug for 6 months. The other three statements are accurate and indicate understanding of TB. Family members should be tested due to repeated exposure to the client. Covering the nose and mouth and placing tissues in plastic bags help prevent transmission of the causative organism. The dietary changes are recommended for clients with TB. **Focus:** Prioritization

19. **Ans: 1** Clients who have recently experienced trauma are at risk for DVT (deep vein thrombosis) and PE. None of the other findings are risk factors for PE. Prolonged immobilization is also a risk factor for DVT and PE, but this period of immobilization is very short. **Focus:** Prioritization

20. **Ans: 4** The LVN/LPN who has been trained to auscultate lung sounds can gather data by routine assessment and observation, under supervision of an RN. Independently evaluating clients and assessing for symptoms of respiratory failure or monitoring and interpreting laboratory values require additional education and skill that are appropriate to the scope of practice for the RN. **Focus:** Delegation/supervision

21. **Ans: 1, 2, 3, 5** While a client is receiving anticoagulation therapy, it is important to avoid trauma to the rectal tissue that could cause bleeding (e.g., avoid rectal temperature taking and enemas). All of the other instructions are appropriate to the care of a client receiving anticoagulation. **Focus:** Delegation/supervision

22. **Ans: 1** A non-rebreather mask can deliver up to 95% oxygen. When the client's oxygenation status does not respond to oxygenation at this high a concentration, this is refractory hypoxemia. Usually at this stage, the client is working very hard to breathe and may go into respiratory arrest unless intubation and mechanical ventilation are provided to decrease the client's work of breathing. **Focus:** Prioritization

23. **Ans: 3** The endotracheal (ET) tube should be marked at the level where it touches the incisor tooth or nares. This mark is used to verify that the tube has not shifted. The other three actions are appropriate after ET tube placement. The priority at this time is to verify that the tube has been correctly placed. **Focus:** Delegation/supervision, prioritization

24. **Ans: 2** The nursing assistant's educational preparation includes taking vital signs, and the experienced nursing assistant would know how to check oxygen saturation by pulse oximetry. Assessing and observing the client, as well as checking ventilator settings, require the additional education and skills of the RN. **Focus:** Delegation/supervision

25. **Ans: 4** Infections are always a threat for the client using a ventilator. The ET tube bypasses the body's normal process of filtering air and provides a direct access for bacteria to the lower parts of the respiratory system. **Focus:** Prioritization

26. **Ans: 3** Confusion in a client this age would be unusual and may be an indication of intracerebral bleeding associated with the enoxaparin use. aPTT testing is not needed for clients receiving fractionated heparin. The right leg symptoms are consistent with a resolving DVT. The presence of ecchymoses may point to a need to do more client teaching about avoiding injury while taking anticoagulants but does not indicate that the physician needs to be called. **Focus:** Prioritization

27. **Ans: 2** Manual ventilation of the client will allow you to deliver an F_{IO_2} of 100%, while you attempt to determine the cause of the high pressure alarm. The client may need reassurance, suctioning, and/or an oral airway, but the first step should be assessment of the reason for the high pressure alarm and resolution of the hypoxemia. **Focus:** Prioritization

28. **Ans: 4** The client's history and symptoms suggest that he may be developing ARDS, which will require intubation and mechanical ventilation. The maximum oxygen delivery with a nasal cannula is an F_{IO_2} of 40%. This is achieved with the O_2 flow at 6 L/minute, so increasing the flow to 10 L/minute will not be helpful. Assisting the client to cough and deep breathe will not improve the lung stiffness that is causing his respiratory distress. Morphine will only decrease the respiratory drive and further contribute to his hypoxemia. **Focus:** Prioritization

29. **Ans: 3** Removal of large quantities of fluid from the pleural space can cause fluid to shift from the circulation into the pleural space, causing hypotension and tachycardia. The client may need IV fluids to correct this. The other data do indicate that the client needs ongoing monitoring and/or interventions, but none of these findings would be unusual for a client with this diagnosis or after this procedure. **Focus:** Prioritization

30. **Ans: 1** Airway clearance techniques are critical for clients with cystic fibrosis (CF) and should take priority over the other activities. The client may need a living will (although the life expectancy for clients with CF is approximately 30 years), but discussion about this may be inappropriate at this time. A private room is not usually required. With increased shortness of breath, it will be more important that the client have frequent respiratory treatments than 8 hours of sleep. **Focus:** Prioritization

Chapter 6: Cardiovascular Problems, pages 37–42

1. **Ans: 2** Cardiac troponins are elevated 3 hours after the onset of ACS (unstable angina or myocardial infarction) and are very specific to cardiac muscle injury or infarction. Although levels of creatine kinase-MB and myoglobin also increase with myocardial infarction, the increases occur later and/or are not as specific to myocardial damage as troponins. Elevated C-reactive protein levels are a risk factor for coronary artery disease, but are not useful in detecting acute injury or infarction. **Focus:** Prioritization

2. **Ans: 4**   Chest pain in a patient having a stress test indicates myocardial ischemia and is an indication to stop the testing to avoid ongoing ischemia, injury, or infarction. Moderate elevations in blood pressure, heart rate, and respiratory rate are a normal response to exercise and are expected during stress testing. **Focus:** Prioritization

3. **Ans: 1**   Because the femoral artery is usually used as the access site during a coronary arteriogram, patients are required to remain on bedrest (with the head only slightly elevated) for several hours after the procedure to avoid arterial bleeding at the site. Even if another arterial site is used, getting patients out of bed only 30 minutes after the procedure would be avoided. The other patient care provided by the LPN/LVN is appropriate. Blood pressure should be checked prior to administration of nitroglycerin. A heart rate increase of more than 20 beats/minute indicates poor cardiac compensation for exercise. Since echocardiography is noninvasive, there is no need to withhold meals before this procedure. **Focus:** Prioritization

4. **Ans: 4**   Lifestyle management, including sodium reduction, is appropriate initial therapy for a patient with stage 1 hypertension and no cardiovascular disease or risk factors. Antihypertensive medications would not be prescribed unless lifestyle changes were attempted for several months without a decrease in blood pressure. This patient's assessment data indicate that she is not overweight and does not drink excessive alcohol, so discussing changes in these risk factors would not be appropriate. **Focus:** Prioritization

5. **Ans: 3**   A persistent and irritating cough (caused by accumulation of bradykinin) is a possible adverse effect of angiotensin-converting enzyme inhibitors such as enalapril and is a common reason for changing to another medication category such as the angiotensin II receptor blockers. The other assessment data indicate a need for more patient teaching and ongoing monitoring, but would not require a change in therapy. **Focus:** Prioritization

6. **Ans: 1**   The patient's major modifiable risk factor is her ongoing smoking. The family history is significant, but changes in behavior will not impact this risk factor. The goal when treating hypertension with medications is reduction of the blood pressure to under 140/90. There is no indication that stress is a risk factor for this patient. **Focus:** Prioritization

7. **Ans: 2**   An RN who worked on a medical-surgical unit would be familiar with left ventricular failure, the administration of IV medications, and the ongoing monitoring for therapeutic and adverse effects of furosemide. The other patients need to be cared for by RNs who are more familiar with the care of patients with acute coronary syndrome and with collaborative treatments such as coronary angioplasty and coronary artery stenting. **Focus:** Assignment

8. **Ans: 4**   Because continuous chest pain lasting for more than 6 hours indicates that reversible myocardial injury has progressed to irreversible myocardial necrosis, fibrinolytic therapy is usually not utilized for patients with chest pain that has lasted for more than 6 hours (in some centers, 12 hours). The other information is also important to communicate, but would not impact the decision about alteplase use. **Focus:** Prioritization

9. **Ans: 1**   Administration of nitroglycerin and appropriate patient monitoring for therapeutic and adverse effects are included in LPN/LVN education and scope of practice. Monitoring of blood pressure, pulse, and oxygen saturation should be delegated to the nursing assistant. Patient teaching requires RN-level education and scope of practice. **Focus:** Delegation

10. **Ans: 2**   The priority for a patient with unstable angina or myocardial infarction is treatment of pain. It is important to remember to assess vital signs prior to administering sublingual nitroglycerin. The other activities also should be accomplished rapidly, but are not as high a priority. **Focus:** Prioritization

11. **Ans: 3**   The best option in this situation is to educate the patient about the purpose of the docusate sodium (to counteract the negative effects of immobility and narcotic use on peristalsis). Charting the medication as "refused" or telling the patient that he should take the docusate sodium simply because it was ordered are possible actions, but not as appropriate as patient education. It is illegal to administer a medication to a patient who is unwilling to take it, unless someone else has health care power of attorney and has authorized the medication. **Focus:** Prioritization

12. **Ans: 4**   The goal in pain management for the patient who is having an AMI is to completely eliminate the pain. Even pain rated at a level 1/10 should be treated with additional morphine sulfate (although possibly a lower dose). The other data indicate a need for ongoing assessment for the possible adverse effects of hypotension, respiratory depression, and dizziness, but do not require further action at this time. **Focus:** Prioritization

13. **Ans: 2**   For behavior to change, the patient must be aware of the need to make changes. This response acknowledges the patient's statement and asks for further clarification. This will give you more information about the patient's feelings, current diet, and activity levels and may increase the willingness to learn. The other responses (while possibly accurate) indicate an intention to teach whether the patient is ready or not and are not likely to lead to changes in patient lifestyle. **Focus:** Prioritization

14. **Ans: 3**   Hyperkalemia is a common adverse effect of both angiotensin-converting enzyme inhibitors and potassium-sparing diuretics. The other laboratory values may be affected by these medications, but are not as likely or as potentially life-threatening. **Focus:** Prioritization

15. **Ans: 1**   The first priority for an ambulating patient who is dizzy is to prevent falls, which could lead to serious injury. The other actions are also appropriate, but not as high a priority. **Focus:** Prioritization

16. **Ans: 1**   Because TEE is performed after the throat is numbed using a topical anesthetic and possibly intravenous sedation, it is important that the patient be NPO for at least 4 to 6 hours prior to the test. The other actions also will need to be accomplished for the TEE, but will not affect how quickly the examination can be scheduled. **Focus:** Prioritization

17. **Ans: 4**   The most common complication after a coronary arteriogram is hemorrhage and the earliest indication of hemorrhage is an increase in heart rate. The other data may also indicate a need for ongoing assessment, but the increase in heart rate is of most concern. **Focus:** Prioritization

18. **Ans: 1**   Measurement of ankle and brachial blood pressures for ankle-brachial index calculation is within the nursing assistant's scope of practice. Calculation of

the ankle-brachial index and any referrals or discussion with the patient are the responsibility of the supervising RN. The other examinations require more complex assessment or patient teaching, which should be done by an experienced RN. **Focus:** Delegation

19. **Ans: 2** The new RN's education and hospital orientation would have included safe administration of IV medications. The preceptor will be responsible for supervision of the new graduate in assessments and patient care. The other patients require more complex assessment or patient teaching by an RN with experience in caring for patients with these diagnoses. **Focus:** Assignment

20. **Ans: 3** Premature ventricular contractions (PVCs) occurring in the setting of acute myocardial injury or infarction can lead to ventricular tachycardia and/or ventricular fibrillation (cardiac arrest), so rapid treatment is necessary. The other patients also have dysrhythmias, which will require further assessment but are not as immediately life-threatening as the PVCs in the setting of myocardial infarction. **Focus:** Prioritization

21. **Ans: 1** The only effective treatment for ventricular fibrillation is defibrillation. If defibrillation is unsuccessful at converting the patient into a perfusing rhythm, CPR should be initiated. Administration of medications and intubation are later interventions. Determination of which of these interventions will be used first depends on other factors, such as whether an IV line is available. **Focus:** Prioritization

22. **Ans: 4** When therapy with carvedilol is started for patients with heart failure, it is expected that their heart failure symptoms will initially become worse for a few weeks, so the increased fatigue, dyspnea, weight gain, and crackles do not indicate a need to discontinue the medication at this time. However, the slow heart rate does require further follow-up, since bradycardia may progress to more serious dysrhythmias such as heart block. **Focus:** Prioritization

23. **Ans: 2** The patient's symptoms indicate acute hypoxia, so immediate further assessments (such as oxygen saturation, neurologic status monitoring, and breath sounds) are indicated. The other patients also should be assessed soon, because they are likely to require nursing actions such as medication administration and teaching but are not as acutely ill as the dyspneic patient. **Focus:** Prioritization

24. **Ans: 2** LPN/LVN education and scope of practice include data collection such as listening to lung sounds and checking for peripheral edema. Weighing the residents should be delegated to nursing assistants. Reviewing medications with residents and planning appropriate activity levels are nursing actions that require RN-level education and scope of practice. **Focus:** Delegation

25. **Ans: 3** The patient's visual disturbances may be a sign of digoxin toxicity. The nurse should notify the physician and obtain an order for a digoxin level. An irregular pulse is expected with atrial fibrillation; there are no contraindications to taking digoxin with food; and crackles that clear with coughing are indicative of atelectasis, not worsening heart failure. **Focus:** Prioritization

26. **Ans: 2,4,3,1** The primary goal is to decrease the cardiac ischemia that is the likely cause of the patient's tachycardia. This would be most rapidly accomplished by decreasing the workload of the heart and administering supplemental oxygen. Changes in blood pressure indicate the impact of the tachycardia on cardiac output and tissue perfusion. Finally, the physician should be notified about the patient's response to activity since changes in therapy may be indicated. **Focus:** Prioritization

27. **Ans: 3** The patient's symptoms indicate that acute arterial occlusion has occurred. Because it is important to return blood flow to the foot rapidly, the physician should be notified immediately so that interventions such as fibrinolytic therapy, balloon angioplasty, or surgery can be initiated. Changing the position of the foot and improving blood oxygen saturation will not improve oxygen delivery to the foot. The patient's vital signs are not indicators of the severity of the problem. **Focus:** Prioritization

28. **Ans: 4** Assisting with hygiene is included in the role and education for nursing assistants. Data collection or assessment about perfusion to the foot and patient teaching are appropriate activities for licensed nursing staff members. **Focus:** Delegation

29. **Ans: 1** Elevated blood pressure in the immediate post-operative period puts stress on the graft suture line and could lead to graft rupture and/or hemorrhage, so it is important to lower the blood pressure quickly. The other data also indicate the need for ongoing assessments and possible interventions, but do not pose an immediate threat to the patient's hemodynamic stability. **Focus:** Prioritization

30. **Ans: 3** Development of plans for patient care or teaching requires RN level education and is the responsibility of the RN. Wound care, medication administration, assisting with ambulation, and reinforcing previously taught information are activities that can be delegated to other nursing personnel, under the supervision of the RN. **Focus:** Delegation

Chapter 7: Hematologic Problems, pages 43–47

1. **Ans: 1** An elevation in white blood cells may indicate that the client has an infection, which would likely require rescheduling of the surgical procedure. The other values are slightly abnormal, but would not be likely to cause post-operative problems for a knee arthroscopy. **Focus:** Prioritization

2. **Ans: 3** Normal saline, an isotonic solution, should be used when priming the IV line to avoid causing hemolysis of RBCs. Ideally, blood products should be infused as soon as possible after they are obtained; however, a 20-minute delay would not be unsafe. Large-gauge IV catheters are preferable for blood administration; if a smaller catheter must be used, normal saline may be used to dilute the RBCs. Although it is appropriate to instruct clients to notify the nurse if symptoms of a transfusion reaction such as shortness of breath or chest pain occur, it will cause unnecessary anxiety to indicate that a serious reaction is likely to occur. **Focus:** Prioritization

3. **Ans: 4** Hypoxia and deoxygenation of the red blood cells are the most common cause of sickling, so administration of oxygen is the priority intervention here. Pain control and hydration are also important interventions for this client and should be accomplished rapidly. Vaccination may help prevent future sickling episodes by decreasing the risk of infection, but it will

not help with the current sickling crisis. **Focus:** Prioritization

4. **Ans: 1**   An experienced nursing assistant would have been taught how to obtain a stool specimen for the Hemoccult slide test, because this is a common screening test for hospitalized clients. Having the client sign an informed consent should be done by the physician who will be doing the colonoscopy. Administration of medications and checking for allergies are within the scope of practice for licensed nursing staff. **Focus:** Delegation

5. **Ans: 3**   A nurse who works in the PACU will be familiar with the monitoring needed for a client who has just returned from a procedure like a colonoscopy, which requires conscious sedation. The other clients require more experience with various types of hematologic disorders and would be better to assign to nursing staff who regularly work on the medical-surgical unit. **Focus:** Assignment

6. **Ans: 1**   Clients with pancytopenia are at higher risk for infection. The client with digoxin toxicity presents the least risk of infecting the new client. Viral pneumonia, shingles, and cellulitis are infectious processes. **Focus:** Prioritization

7. **Ans: 2**   The joint pain that occurs in sickle cell crisis is caused by obstruction of blood flow by the sickled red blood cells. The appropriate therapy for this client would be application of moist heat to the joints to cause vasodilation and improve circulation. Because control of pain is a priority during sickle cell crisis, encouraging the client to use the PCA is an appropriate therapy. While infection control is important in preventing and treating sickle cell crisis, there is no need to restrict all visitors or to check the temperature every 2 hours. **Focus:** Prioritization

8. **Ans: 3**   Because aspirin will decrease platelet aggregation, clients with thrombocytopenia should not use aspirin routinely. Client teaching about this should be included in the care plan. Bruising is consistent with the client's admission problem of thrombocytopenia. Soft, dark brown stools indicate that there is no frank blood in the bowel movements. A decrease in appetite is common with chemotherapy, and more assessment is indicated. **Focus:** Prioritization

9. **Ans: 2**   When a hemophiliac client is at high risk for bleeding, for example, after a motor vehicle accident, the priority intervention is to maximize the availability of clotting factors. The other orders also should be implemented rapidly, but do not have as high a priority. **Focus:** Prioritization

10. **Ans: 1**   Clients taking warfarin are advised to avoid making sudden diet changes, because changing the oral intake of foods high in vitamin K (such as green leafy vegetables and some fruits) will have an impact on the effectiveness of the medication. The other statements suggest that further teaching may be indicated, but more assessment for teaching needs is indicated first. **Focus:** Prioritization

11. **Ans: 3**   Because the decrease in oxygen saturation will have the greatest immediate effect on all body systems, improvement in oxygenation should be the priority goal of care. The other data also indicate the need for rapid intervention, but improvement of oxygenation is the most urgent need. **Focus:** Prioritization

12. **Ans: 3**   More assessment about what the client means is needed before any interventions can be planned or

implemented. All of the other statements indicate a conclusion that the client is afraid of dying of Hodgkin's disease. **Focus:** Prioritization

13. **Ans: 4**   Any temperature elevation in a neutropenic client may indicate the presence of a life-threatening infection, so actions such as blood cultures and antibiotic administration should be initiated quickly. The other clients need to be assessed as soon as possible, but are not critically ill. **Focus:** Prioritization

14. **Ans: 2**   Nursing assistant education includes routine nursing skills such as assessment of vital signs. Evaluation, baseline assessment of client abilities, and nutrition planning are roles appropriate to RN practice. **Focus:** Delegation

15. **Ans: 3**   The client's symptoms indicate that a transfusion reaction may be occurring, so the first action should be to stop the transfusion. Chills are an indication of a febrile reaction, so warming the client is not appropriate. Checking the client's temperature and administration of oxygen are also appropriate actions if a transfusion reaction is suspected; however, stopping the transfusion is the priority. **Focus:** Prioritization

16. **Ans: 1**   Subcutaneous administration of epoetin is within the LPN/LVN scope of practice. The other clients require skills (blood transfusion and client teaching about phlebotomy and bone marrow aspiration) that are more appropriate to RN-level practice. **Focus:** Assignment

17. **Ans: 4**   The lack of plantar flexion may indicate spinal cord compression, which should be evaluated and treated immediately by the physician to prevent further loss of function. While chronic bone pain, hyperuricemia, and the presence of Bence-Jones protein in the urine all are typical of multiple myeloma and do require assessment and/or treatment; the loss of motor or sensory function is an emergency. **Focus:** Prioritization

18. **Ans: 2**   Because the spleen has an important role in the phagocytosis of microorganisms, the client is at higher risk for severe infection after a splenectomy. Medical therapy, such as antibiotic administration, is usually indicated for any symptoms of infection. The other information also indicates the need for more assessment and intervention, but prevention and treatment of infection are the highest priorities for this client. **Focus:** Prioritization

19. **Ans: 3**   Infusion of IV fluids is included in RN education, and the new RN would also have had experience with this as part of an orientation to the medical unit. Administration of potent immunosuppressive medications, assessment for subtle indications of infection, and client teaching are more complex tasks that should be delegated to more experienced RN staff members. **Focus:** Delegation

20. **Ans: 3**   Because many aspects of nursing care need to be modified to prevent infection when a client has a low ANC, care should be provided by the staff member with the most experience with neutropenic clients. The other staff members have the education required to care for this client, but are not as clinically experienced. When making acute care client assignments for LPN staff members, they must work under the supervision of an RN. The LPN in this case would report to the RN assigned to the client. **Focus:** Assignment

21. **Ans: 4**   The neutropenic client is at increased risk for infection, so the LTC charge nurse needs to know

this in order to make decisions about the client room assignment and to plan care. The other information also will impact on planning for client care, but the charge nurse needs the information about neutropenia before the client is transferred. **Focus:** Prioritization

22. **Ans: 1**   Fatal hyperkalemia may be caused by tumor lysis syndrome, a potentially serious consequence of chemotherapy in acute leukemia. The other symptoms also indicate a need for further assessment or interventions, but are not as critical as the elevated potassium level. **Focus:** Prioritization

23. **Ans: 2**   A non-tender swelling in this area (or near any lymph node) may indicate that the client has developed lymphoma, a possible adverse effect of immunosuppressive therapy. The client should receive further evaluation immediately. The other symptoms may also indicate side effects of cyclosporine (gingival hyperplasia, nausea, paresthesia), but do not indicate the need for immediate action. **Focus:** Prioritization

24. **Ans: 4**   Skin care is included in nursing assistant education and job description. Assessment and client teaching are more complex tasks that should be delegated to registered nurses. Use of lotions to the irradiated area is usually avoided during radiation therapy. **Focus:** Delegation

25. **Ans: 1**   The newly admitted client should be assessed first, because the baseline assessment and plan of care need to be completed. The other clients also need assessments or interventions, but do not need immediate nursing care. **Focus:** Prioritization

Chapter 8: Neurologic Problems, pages 49–54

1. **Ans: 1**   The priority for interdisciplinary care for the patient experiencing a migraine headache is pain management. All of the other nursing diagnoses are accurate, but none of them is as urgent as the issue of pain, which is often incapacitating. **Focus:** Prioritization

2. **Ans: 1, 2, 3, 4, 5**   Medications such as estrogen supplements may actually trigger a migraine headache attack. All of the other statements are accurate. **Focus:** Prioritization

3. **Ans: 3**   Taking vital signs is within the education and scope of practice for a nursing assistant. The nurse should perform neurologic checks and document the seizure. Patients with seizures should not be restrained; however, the nurse may guide the patient's movements as necessary. **Focus:** Delegation/supervision

4. **Ans: 2**   The LPN/LVN can set up the equipment for oxygen and suctioning. The RN should perform the complete initial assessment. Padded side rails are controversial in terms of whether they actually provide safety and may embarrass the patient and family. Tongue blades should not be at the bedside and should never be inserted into the patient's mouth after a seizure begins. **Focus:** Delegation/supervision

5. **Ans: 4**   A patient with a seizure disorder should not take over-the-counter medications without consulting with the physician first. The other three statements are appropriate teaching points for patients with seizure disorders and their families. **Focus:** Delegation/supervision

6. **Ans: 3**   The nursing assistant should assist the patient with morning care as needed, but the goal is to keep this patient as independent and mobile as possible. The patient should be encouraged to perform as much morning care as possible. Assisting the patient to

ambulate, reminding the patient not to look at his feet (to prevent falls), and encouraging the patient to feed himself are all appropriate to the goal of maintaining independence. **Focus:** Delegation/supervision

7. **Ans: 1**   Exercises are used to strengthen the back, relieve pressure on compressed nerves and protect the back from re-injury. Ice, heat, and firm mattresses are appropriate interventions for back pain. People with chronic back pain should avoid wearing high-heeled shoes at all times. **Focus:** Prioritization

8. **Ans: 2**   These signs and symptoms are characteristic of autonomic dysreflexia, a neurologic emergency that must be promptly treated to prevent a hypertensive stroke. The cause of this syndrome is noxious stimuli, most often a distended bladder or constipation, so checking for poor catheter drainage, bladder distention, or fecal impaction is the first action that should be taken. Adjusting the room temperature may be helpful, since too cool a temperature in the room may contribute to the problem. Tylenol will not decrease the autonomic dysreflexia that is causing the patient's headache. Notification of the physician may be necessary if nursing actions do not resolve symptoms. **Focus:** Prioritization

9. **Ans: 2**   The new graduate RN who is oriented to the unit should be assigned stable, non-complex patients, such as the patient with stroke. The patient with Parkinson's disease needs assistance with bathing, which is best delegated to the nursing assistant. The patient being transferred to the nursing home and the newly admitted SCI should be assigned to experienced nurses. **Focus:** Assignment

10. **Ans: 4**   The first priority for the patient with an SCI is assessing respiratory patterns and ensuring an adequate airway. The patient with a high cervical injury is at risk for respiratory compromise because the spinal nerves (C3-5) innervate the phrenic nerve, which controls the diaphragm. The other assessments are also necessary, but not as high priority. **Focus:** Prioritization

11. **Ans: 2**   The nursing assistant's training and education include taking and recording patient's vital signs. The nursing assistant may assist with turning and repositioning the patient and may remind the patient to cough and deep breathe but does not teach the patient how to perform these actions. Assessing and monitoring patients require additional education and are appropriate to the scope of practice for professional nurses. **Focus:** Delegation/supervision

12. **Ans: 1, 2, 4, 5**   All of the strategies, except straight catheterization, may stimulate voiding in patients with SCI. Intermittent bladder catheterization can be used to empty the patient's bladder, but it will not stimulate voiding. **Focus:** Prioritization

13. **Ans: 1, 3, 4**   Checking and observing for signs of pressure or infection are within the scope of practice of the LPN/LVN. The LPN/LVN also has the appropriate skills for cleaning the halo insertion sites with hydrogen peroxide. Neurologic examination requires additional education and skill appropriate to the professional RN. **Focus:** Delegation/supervision

14. **Ans: 3**   The patient's statement indicates impairment of adjustment to the limitations of the injury and indicates the need for additional counseling, teaching, and support. The other three nursing diagnoses may be appropriate to the patient with SCI, but they are not related to the patient's statement. **Focus:** Prioritization

15. **Ans: 2**   The traveling nurse is relatively new to neurologic nursing and should be assigned patients whose conditions are stable and not complex. The newly diagnosed patient will need lots of teaching and support. The patient with respiratory distress will need frequent assessments and may need to be transferred to the ICU. The patient with C4 SCI is at risk for respiratory arrest. All three of these patients should be assigned to nurses experienced in neurologic nursing care. **Focus:** Assignment

16. **Ans: 4**   At this time, based on the patient's statement, the priority is Self-Care Deficit related to fatigue after physical therapy. The other three nursing diagnoses are appropriate to a patient with MS, but they are not related to the patient's statement. **Focus:** Prioritization

17. **Ans: 4**   The priority interventions for the patient with GBS are aimed at maintaining adequate respiratory function. These patients are at risk for respiratory failure, which is urgent. The other findings are important and should be reported to the nurse, but they are not life-threatening. **Focus:** Prioritization, delegation/supervision

18. **Ans: 2**   The changes that the nursing assistant is reporting are characteristic of myasthenic crisis, which often follows some type of infection. The patient is at risk for inadequate respiratory function. In addition to notifying the physician, the nurse should carefully monitor the patient's respiratory status. The patient may need intubation and mechanical ventilation. The nurse would notify the physician before giving the suppository because there may be orders for cultures before giving acetaminophen. This patient's vital signs need to be re-checked sooner than 1 hour. Rescheduling the physical therapy can be delegated to the unit clerk and is not urgent. **Focus:** Prioritization

19. **Ans: 3**   Alteplase is a clot buster. With a patient who has experienced hemorrhagic stroke, there is already bleeding into the brain. A drug like alteplase can worsen the bleeding. The other statements are also accurate about use of alteplase, but they are not pertinent to this patient's diagnosis. **Focus:** Prioritization

20. **Ans: 1**   Patients with right cerebral hemisphere stroke often present with neglect syndrome. They lean to the left and when asked, respond that they believe they are sitting up straight. They often neglect the left side of their bodies and ignore food on the left side of their food trays. The nurse would need to remind the student of this phenomenon and discuss the appropriate interventions. **Focus:** Delegation/supervision

21. **Ans: 1, 2, 3**   The experienced nursing assistant would know how to reposition the patient and how to reapply compression boots, and would remind the patient to perform activities he has been taught to perform. Assessing for redness and swelling (signs of deep venous thrombosis [DVT]) requires additional education and skill appropriate to the professional nurse. **Focus:** Delegation/supervision

22. **Ans: 1**   Positioning the patient in a sitting position decreases the risk of aspiration. The nursing assistant is not trained to assess gag or swallowing reflexes. The patient should not be rushed during feeding. A patient who needs to be suctioned between bites of food is not handling secretions and is at risk for aspiration. This patient should be assessed further before feeding. **Focus:** Delegation/supervision

23. **Ans: 2**   Untreated bacterial meningitis has a mortality rate approaching 100%, so rapid antibiotic treatment is essential. The other interventions will help reduce CNS stimulation and irritation, and should be implemented as soon as possible. **Focus:** Prioritization

24. **Ans: 1**   Meningococcal meningitis is spread through contact with respiratory secretions so use of a mask and gown is required to prevent spread of the infection to staff members or other patients. The other actions may not be appropriate, but they do not require intervention as rapidly. The presence of a family member at the bedside may decrease patient confusion and agitation. Patients with hyperthermia frequently complain of feeling chilled, but warming the patient is not an appropriate intervention. Checking the pupil response to light is appropriate, but it is not needed every 30 minutes and is uncomfortable for a patient with photophobia. **Focus:** Prioritization

25. **Ans: 2**   Administration of medications is included in LPN education and scope of practice. Collection of data about the seizure activity may be accomplished by an LPN/LVN who observes initial seizure activity. An LPN/LVN would know to call the supervising RN immediately if a patient started to seize. Documentation of the seizure, patient teaching, and planning of care are complex activities that require RN level education and scope of practice. **Focus:** Delegation

26. **Ans: 3**   The priority action during a generalized tonic-clonic seizure is to protect the airway. Administration of lorazepam should be the next action, since it will act rapidly to control the seizure. Although oxygen may be useful during the postictal phase, the hypoxemia during tonic-clonic seizures is caused by apnea. Checking the level of consciousness is not appropriate during the seizure, because generalized tonic-clonic seizures are associated with a loss of consciousness. **Focus:** Prioritization

27. **Ans: 2**   Leukopenia is a serious adverse effect of phenytoin and would require discontinuation of the medication. The other data indicate a need for further assessment and/or patient teaching, but will not require a change in medical treatment for the seizures. **Focus:** Prioritization

28. **Ans: 4**   Urinary tract infections are a frequent complication in patients with multiple sclerosis because of the effect on bladder function. The elevated temperature and flank pain suggest that this patient may have pyelonephritis. The physician should be notified immediately so that antibiotic therapy can be started quickly. The other patients should be assessed soon, but do not have needs as urgent as this patient. **Focus:** Prioritization

29. **Ans: 1, 3, 5**   NA education and scope of practice includes taking pulse and blood pressure measurements. In addition, NAs can reinforce previous teaching or skills taught by the RN or other disciplines, such as speech or physical therapists. Evaluation of patient response to medications and development and individualizing the plan of care require RN-level education and scope of practice. **Focus:** Delegation

30. **Ans: 1**   LPN education and team leader responsibilities include checking for the therapeutic and adverse effects of medications. Changes in the residents' memory would be communicated to the RN supervisor, who is responsible for overseeing the plan of care for each resident. Assessment for changes on the Mini-Mental State Examination and developing the plan of care are RN responsibilities. Assisting residents with personal

care and hygiene would be delegated to nursing assistants working at the LTC facility. **Focus:** Delegation

31. **Ans: 2** The husband's statement about lack of sleep and anxiety over whether the patient is receiving the correct medications are behaviors that support this diagnosis. There is no evidence that the patient's cardiac output is decreased. The husband's statements about how he monitors the patient and his concern with medication administration indicate that the Risk for Ineffective Therapeutic Regimen Management and falls are not priorities at this time. **Focus:** Prioritization

32. **Ans: 1** The inability to recognize a family member is a new neurologic deficit for this patient, and indicates a possible increase in intracranial pressure (ICP). This change should be communicated to the physician immediately so that treatment can be initiated. The continued headache also indicates that the ICP may be elevated, but it is not a new problem. The glucose elevation and weight gain are common adverse effects of dexamethasone that may require treatment, but they are not emergencies. **Focus:** Prioritization

33. **Ans: 2** The patient's history and assessment data indicate that he may have a chronic subdural hematoma. The priority goal is to obtain a rapid diagnosis and send the patient to surgery to have the hematoma evacuated. The other interventions also should be implemented as soon as possible, but the initial nursing activities should be directed toward treatment of any intracranial lesion. **Focus:** Prioritization

34. **Ans: 3** This patient is the most stable of the patients listed. An RN from the medical unit would be familiar with administration of IV antibiotics. The other patients require assessments and care from RNs more experienced in caring for patients with neurologic diagnoses. **Focus:** Assignment

Chapter 9: Visual and Auditory Problems, pages 55–58

1. **Ans: 3** If the client is wearing contact lenses, the lenses may be causing the symptoms and removing them prevents further eye irritation or damage. Policies on giving telephone advice will vary between institutions, and knowledge of your facility policy is essential. The other options may be appropriate, but you should gather additional information before suggesting anything else. **Focus:** Prioritization

2. **Ans: 3** Most (90%) accidental eye injuries could be prevented by wearing protective eyewear for sports and hazardous work. Other options should be considered in the overall prevention of injuries, but have less impact. **Focus:** Prioritization

3. **Ans: 1, 3** Post-operative instructions and home health referrals should be done by an experienced nurse who can give specific details and specialized information for follow-up eye care. The principles of eye pad and shield application and of teaching the administration of eye drops are basic procedures that should be familiar to all nurses. **Focus:** Assignment

4. **Ans: 6, 2, 5, 4, 3, 1** Have the client sit with head hyperextended. Pulling down the lower conjunctival sac creates a small pocket for the drops. Stabilizing the hand prevents accidentally poking the client's eye. Having the client look up prevents the drop from falling on the cornea and stimulating the blink reflex. When the client gently moves the eye, the medication is distrib-

uted. Pressing on the lacrimal duct prevents systemic absorption. **Focus:** Prioritization

5. **Ans: 2, 3, 4** Administering medications and reviewing and demonstrating standard procedures with predictable outcomes in non-complex cases are within the scope of the LPN/LVN. Assessing systemic manifestations and behaviors is the responsibility of the RN. **Focus:** Delegation

6. **Ans: 2** Despite the fact that the child is still screaming, the mother must continue to irrigate the eyes for at least 20 minutes or until the emergency medical service arrives. Another adult, if present, should call Poison Control and 911. **Focus:** Prioritization

7. **Ans: 1** Warm compresses will usually provide relief. If the problem persists, eyelid scrubs and antibiotic drops would be appropriate. The ophthalmologist could be consulted, but other providers such as the family doctor or the nurse practitioner could give a prescription for antibiotics. **Focus:** Prioritization

8. **Ans: 4** A curtain-like shadow is a symptom of retinal detachment, which is an emergency situation. Change in color vision is a symptom of cataract. Crusty drainage is associated with conjunctivitis. Increased lacrimation is associated with many eye irritants, such as allergies, contact lenses, or foreign bodies. **Focus:** Prioritization

9. **Ans: 2** Assisting the client to ambulate in the hall is within the scope of the nursing assistant. Dealing with the client's emotional state, orienting the client to the room, and encouraging independence require formative evaluation to gauge readiness, and these activities should be the responsibility of the RN. **Focus:** Delegation

10. **Ans: 4** Intense pain may signal hemorrhage, infection, or increased ocular pressure. A scratchy sensation and loss of depth perception with the patch in place are not uncommon. Adequate vision may not return for 24 hours. **Focus:** Prioritization

11. **Ans: 1** African Americans have the greatest risk of developing glaucoma. Current recommendations are eye examinations every 2–4 years for people age 40–64 and every 1–2 years for those older than 65. African Americans at all ages need more frequent examinations. **Focus:** Prioritization

12. **Ans: 4** All beta-adrenergic blockers are contraindicated in bradycardia. Alpha-adrenergic agents can cause tachycardia and hypertension. Carbonic anhydrase inhibitors should not be given to clients with rheumatoid arthritis who are taking high doses of aspirin. **Focus:** Prioritization

13. **Ans: 1, 2, 3** Irrigating the ear, giving medication, and reminding the client about post-operative instructions that were given by the RN are within the scope of practice of the LPN/LVN. Counseling clients is the responsibility of the RN. **Focus:** Delegation

14. **Ans: 1** Gentamicin is potentially ototoxic. The prescribing physician should be notified so that the drug can be discontinued. The other options are not associated with hearing problems. **Focus:** Prioritization

15. **Ans: 2** This client has a hearing loss, and a referral for a hearing aid or rehabilitation program would be the first step to correct the physical problem. The other diagnoses are pertinent if the hearing loss continues to interfere with her quality of life. **Focus:** Prioritization

16. **Ans: 3** A bulging red or blue tympanic membrane is a possible sign of otitis media or perforation. Other signs are considered normal anatomy. **Focus:** Prioritization

17. **Ans: 3** Vertigo without hearing loss should be further assessed for nonvestibular causes, such as cardiovascular or metabolic. The other options are more associated with inner ear or labyrinthine causes. **Focus:** Prioritization

18. **Ans: 1. MD, 2. NA, 3. LPN/LVN, 4. MD, 5. RN** The physician is responsible for determining medical diagnosis and for explaining outcomes and risks of surgical procedures. A physical therapist will teach and evaluate movement and ambulation techniques; however, the nursing assistant (under supervision) is able to help clients with routine ambulation and position changes. The LPN/LVN is qualified to give medications and works under the supervision of the RN. The RN should assess the client to identify situations associated with vertigo. **Focus:** Assignment

19. **Ans: 3** Heavy lifting should be strictly avoided after stapedectomy for at least 3 weeks. Water in the ear and air travel should be avoided for at least 1 week. Coughing and sneezing should be performed with the mouth open to prevent increased pressure. **Focus:** Prioritization

20. **Ans: 3, 5, 4, 2, 1** The type of foreign body (e.g., insect, bean, bead) will determine the next steps. If there is a live insect, instill oil. Vegetable or insect matter will swell if water is used for irrigation. Tightly wedged objects like beads are difficult to flush. If perforation is suspected or if the object is not easily removed, the nurse should not attempt irrigation or instillation. Check for trauma after the object is removed. If trauma occurred, the client should be referred for antibiotics to prevent infection. **Focus:** Prioritization

Chapter 10: Musculoskeletal Problems, pages 59–62

1. **Ans: 4** Assisting with activities of daily living is within the scope of the nursing assistant's practice. The other three interventions require additional educational preparation and are within the scope of practice of licensed nurses. **Focus:** Delegation/supervision

2. **Ans: 1, 2, 3, 5** The purpose of the teaching is to help the patient prevent falls. The hip protector can prevent hip fractures if the patient falls. Throw rugs and obstacles in the home increase the risk of falls. Patients who are tired are also more likely to fall. Exercise helps to strengthen muscles and improve coordination. **Focus:** Prioritization

3. **Ans: 2** Platybasia (basilar skull invagination) causes brain stem manifestations that threaten life. Patients with Paget's disease are usually short and often have bowing of the long bones that results in asymmetric knees or elbow deformities. Their skull is typically soft, thick, and enlarged. **Focus:** Prioritization.

4. **Ans: 3** Application of heat, not ice, is the appropriate measure to help reduce the patient's pain. Ibuprofen is useful to manage mild to moderate pain. Exercise prescribed by the PT is non-impact in nature and provides strengthening for the patient. A diet rich in calcium promotes bone health. **Focus:** Delegation/supervision

5. **Ans: 4** The PACU nurse is very familiar with the assessment skills necessary to monitor a newly post-operative patient. The other patients need care from nurses familiar with musculoskeletal-related nursing care, to provide teaching, assessment, and report to the long-term care facility. **Focus:** Assignment

6. **Ans: 1** An elevated temperature indicates infection and inflammation. This patient needs IV antibiotic therapy. The other vital signs are normal or high normal results. **Focus:** Delegation/supervision

7. **Ans: Clear, Concise, Correct, Complete** The 4 Cs of communication help the nurse ensure that the nursing assistant understands what is being said and does not confuse the nurse's directions; that directions are according to policies, procedures, job descriptions, and the law; and that the nursing assistant has all the information to complete the tasks assigned. **Focus:** Delegation/supervision.

8. **Ans: 3** Placing a splint for the first time is appropriate to the scope of practice for physical therapists. Assessing and testing for paresthesia are not within the scope of practice for nursing assistants. Assistance with activities of daily living is within the scope of practice for a nursing assistant. **Focus:** Delegation/supervision

9. **Ans: 3** When a patient with CTS has a splint used for immobilization of the wrist, it is placed either in the neutral position or in slight extension. The other interventions are correct and are within the scope of practice for a nursing assistant. Nursing assistants may remind patients about elements of their care plans such as avoiding heavy lifting. **Focus:** Delegation/supervision.

10. **Ans: 1** Post-operative pain and numbness occur for a longer period of time with endoscopic carpal tunnel release than with the open procedure. Patients often need assistance post-operatively, even after they are discharged. The dressing from the endoscopic procedure is usually very small and there should not be a lot of drainage. **Focus:** Prioritization

11. **Ans: 1, 2, 3, 5** Post-operatively, patients with OCTR surgery have pain and numbness. Their discomfort may last for weeks to months. All of the other directions are appropriate to the post-operative care of this patient. It is important to monitor for drainage, tightness, and neurovascular changes. Raising the hand/wrist above the heart reduces the swelling from surgery, and this is often done for several days. **Focus:** Assignment, delegation/supervision

12. **Ans: 2** Hand movements, including heavy lifting, may be restricted for 4–6 weeks after surgery. Patients experience discomfort for weeks to months after surgery. The surgery is not always a cure. In some cases, CTS may recur months to years after surgery. **Focus:** Prioritization

13. **Ans: 1** Ibuprofen can cause abdominal discomfort or pain and gastrointestinal ulceration. In such cases, it should be given with meals or milk. Removal of throw rugs helps prevent falls. Range-of-motion exercises and rest are important strategies for coping with osteoporosis. **Focus:** Prioritization.

14. **Ans: 2** Fat embolism syndrome is a serious complication that is often the result of fractures of long bones. The earliest manifestation of this is altered mental status caused by low arterial oxygen level. The nurse would want to know about and treat the pain, but it is not life threatening. The nurse would also want to know about the blood pressure and that the patient voided; however, neither of these pieces of information is urgent. **Focus:** Prioritizaton, delegation/supervision

15. **Ans: 3** The patient with the tight cast is at risk for circulation impairment and peripheral nerve damage. While all of the other patients' concerns are important and the nurse will want to see them as soon as pos-

sible, none of their concerns is urgent. **Focus:** Prioritization

16. **Ans: 3**   When the weights are resting on the floor, they are not exerting pulling force to provide reduction and alignment, or to prevent muscle spasm. The weights should always hang freely. Attending to the weights may reduce the patient's pain and spasm. With skeletal pins, a small amount of clear fluid drainage is expected. It is important to inspect the traction system after a patient changes position because position changes may alter the traction. **Focus:** Delegation/supervision, prioritization

17. **Ans: 1**   Moving from a lying position to a sitting position, then a standing position allows the patient to establish balance prior to standing. Administering pain medication prior to exercising decreases pain with exercise. Explanations about the purpose of the exercise program and proper use of crutches are appropriate interventions with this patient. **Focus:** Delegation/supervision

18. **Ans: 2**   Monitoring for sufficient tissue perfusion is the priority at this time. Phantom pain is a concern, but is more common in patients with above-the-knee amputations. Early ambulation is a goal, but at this time, the patient is more likely to be engaged in muscle-strengthening exercises. Elevation of the residual limb on a pillow is controversial because it may promote knee flexion contracture. **Focus:** Delegation/supervision

19. **Ans: 1**   There are three theories being researched with regard to PLP. The peripheral nervous system theory implies that sensations remain as a result of severing peripheral nerves during the amputation. The central nervous system theory states that PLP results from a loss of inhibitory signals that are generated through afferent impulses from the amputated limb. The psychological theory helps predict and explain PLP in that stress, anxiety, and depression often trigger or worsen an episode of PLP. **Focus:** Prioritization

20. **Ans: 4**   The patient is indicating an interest in learning about prostheses. The experienced nurse can initiate discussion and begin educating the patient. Certainly the physician can also discuss prostheses with the patient, but the patient's wish to learn should receive a quick response. The nurse can then notify the physician about the patient's request. **Focus:** Delegation/supervision

21. **Ans: 1**   Pressure and pain may be due to increased compartment pressure and indicate the serious complication of acute compartment syndrome. This is urgent. If not treated, cyanosis, tingling, numbness, paresis, and severe pain occur. **Focus:** Prioritization

Chapter 11: Gastrointestinal and Nutritional Problems, pages 63–67

1. **Ans: 2**   The nursing assistant can reinforce dietary and fluid restrictions after the RN has explained the information to the client. It is also possible that the nursing assistant can administer the enema; however, special training is required and policies may vary between institutions. Medication administration should be performed by licensed personnel. **Focus:** Delegation

2. **Ans: 4**   A client with a fractured femur is at risk for fat embolism, so fat emulsion should be used with caution. Vomiting may be a problem if the emulsion is infused too rapidly. TPN is commonly used for gas-

trointestinal obstruction, severe anorexia nervosa, and chronic diarrhea or vomiting. **Focus:** Prioritization

3. **Ans: 3, 5, 2, 1, 4, 6**   The solution should not be cloudy or turbid. Prepare the equipment, by priming the tubing and threading the pump. To prevent infection, use aseptic technique when inserting the connector into the injection cap and connecting the tubing to the central line. Set the pump at the prescribed rate. **Focus:** Prioritization

4. **Ans: 4**   A board-like abdomen with shoulder pain is a symptom of a perforation, which is the most lethal complication of peptic ulcer disease. A burning sensation is a typical complaint, which can be controlled with medications. Projectile vomiting can signal an obstruction. Coffee-ground emesis is typical of slower bleeding and will require diagnostic testing. **Focus:** Prioritization

5. **Ans: 2**   Body dysmorphic disorder is a preoccupation with an imagined physical defect. Corrective surgery can exacerbate this disorder when the client continues to feel dissatisfied with the results. The other criteria are indicators of candidacy for this treatment. **Focus:** Prioritization

6. **Ans: 1, 2, 3**   First, antacids and over-the counter histamine-2 blockers are used. In step two, prescription histamine-2 blockers are prescribed. Finally, proton-pump inhibitors are used. **Focus:** Prioritization

7. **Ans: 3**   Reminding the client to follow through on advice given by the nurse is an appropriate task for the nursing assistant. The RN should take responsibility for teaching rationale and discussing strategies for the treatment plan and assessing client concerns. **Focus:** Delegation

8. **Ans: 1, 2, 6, 3, 5, 4**   Assessment is the first step. Checking for tube placement prevents accidentally instilling feeding/medication into the lungs. The amount of residual volume determines whether the amount of the scheduled feeding is appropriate or whether the physician should be notified. Flushing the tube before and after feeding helps maintain tube patency. **Focus:** Prioritization

9. **Ans: 4**   Nausea and vomiting are common after chemotherapy. Administration of antiemetics and fluid monitoring can be done by an LPN/LVN. The RN should do the pre-operative teaching for the glossectomy client. Clients returning from surgery need extensive assessment. The client with anorexia is showing signs of hypokalemia and is at risk for cardiac dysrhythmias. **Focus:** Assignment

10. **Ans: 3**   The LPN/LVN can assist in the planning of interventions, but the RN should take ultimate responsibility for planning or designing. Obtaining equipment should be delegated to the nursing assistant. Contact physical therapy to set up specialized equipment. **Focus:** Delegation

11. **Ans: 4**   Showing the student how to insert the suppository meets that immediate client need and the student's learning need. The instructor can address the student's fears and long-term learning needs once he/she is aware of the incident. It is preferable that students express fears and learning needs. The other options will discourage the student's future disclosure of clinical limitations and need for additional training. **Focus:** Supervision/assignment

12. **Ans: 3, 1, 7, 5, 2, 4, 6**   Prepare the warm water (cold water can cause cramping) and hang the container at

shoulder height (hanging the container too high or too low will alter the rate of flow). Put on a pair of clean gloves to protect your hands from colostomy secretions. Lubricating the stoma and gently inserting will allow the water to flow into the stoma. A slow and steady flow prevents cramps and spillage. Adequate time allows for complete evacuation. Careful attention to the skin prevents breakdown. **Focus:** Prioritization

13. **Ans: 3** Disconnecting the tube from suction is an appropriate task to delegate. Suction should be reconnected by the nurse, so that correct pressure is checked. If the nursing assistant is permitted to reconnect the tube, the RN is still responsible for checking that the pressure setting is correct. During removal of the tube, there is a potential for aspiration, so the nurse should perform this task. If the tube is dislodged, the nurse should recheck placement before it is secured. **Focus:** Delegation

14. **Ans: 3** The goal of bowel training is to establish a pattern that mimics normal defecation, and many people have the urge to defecate after a meal. If this is not successful, a suppository can be used to stimulate the urge. Incontinence briefs are embarrassing for the client and must be changed frequently to prevent skin breakdown. Routine use of rectal tubes is not recommended because of damage to the mucosa and sphincter tone. **Focus:** Prioritization

15. **Ans: 1** The immediate problem is controlling the diarrhea. Addressing this problem is a step to correcting the nutritional imbalance and decreasing the diarrheal cramping. Self-care and compliance with the treatment plan are important long-term goals that can be addressed when the client is feeling better physically. **Focus:** Prioritization

16. **Ans: 3, 4, 2, 1, 6, 5** Immediate decontamination is appropriate because time can affect viral load. Occupational health will direct the employee in filing the correct forms, getting the appropriate laboratory tests, getting appropriate prophylaxis, and following up on results. **Focus:** Prioritization

17. **Ans: 2, 4, 5, 1, 3, 6** Stay calm and stay with the client. If the client does anything to increase intra-abdominal pressure, the evisceration will worsen. Have a colleague gather supplies and notify the physician. Putting the client in a semi-Fowler's position with knees flexed will decrease the strain on the wound site. Covering the site provides protection of tissue. Monitor vital signs particularly for decrease in blood pressure or increase in pulse. Anticipate and prepare the client for emergency surgery. **Focus:** Prioritization

18. **Ans: 3** RUQ pain is a sign of hemorrhage or bile leak. Ability to void should return within 6 hours post-operatively. Right shoulder pain is related to unabsorbed CO_2 and will resolve by placing the client in the Sims' position. Output that does not equal input after surgery for the first several hours is expected. **Focus:** Prioritization

19. **Ans: 1** The nursing assistant should use infection control precautions for the protection of self, employees, and other clients. Planning and monitoring are RN responsibilities. While the nursing assistants can report valuable information, they should not be responsible for signs and symptoms that can be subtle or hard to detect, such as skin changes. **Focus:** Delegation

20. **Ans: 1** When a client has esophageal varices, the vessels become very fragile and massive hemorrhage can occur. The mortality rate is 30%–50% after an episode

of bleeding. Ascites and edema occur when liver production of albumin fails. Asterixis is a sign of hepatic encephalopathy. **Focus:** Prioritization

21. **Ans: 2** Assisting with procedures in stable clients with predictable outcomes is within the educational scope of the LPN/LVN. Teaching the client about self-care or pathophysiology and evaluating the outcome of interventions are responsibilities of the RN. **Focus:** Delegation

22. **Ans: 1** Distention and rigidity can signal hemorrhage or peritonitis. Physician may also decide that symptoms require a medication to stimulate peristalsis. Absent bowel sounds are expected within the first 24–48 hours. Nausea and vomiting are not uncommon and are usually self-limiting, and a PRN order for an antiemetic is usually part of the routine post-operative orders. Assess the client's reason for pulling tube, and secure as necessary. **Focus:** Prioritization

23. **Ans: 2, 3** Both clients will need frequent pain assessments and medications. Clients with copious diarrhea or vomiting will frequently need enteric isolation. Cancer clients receiving chemotherapy are at risk for immunosuppression and are likely to need reverse isolation. **Focus:** Assignment

24. **Ans: 2** The experienced medical-surgical nurse will know the types of questions that clients generally ask during pre-operative or discharge teaching. The new graduate may have enthusiasm and knowledge, but will lack practical application. SICU nurses are less involved in pre-operative or discharge teaching. LPN/LVNs can do teaching, but their educational scope does not provide for development of teaching materials and strategies. **Focus:** Assignment

25. **Ans: 1, 3, 4, 5** Strangulated intestinal obstruction is a surgical emergency. NG tube is for decompression of the intestine. Abdominal x-ray is the most useful diagnostic aid. IV fluids are needed to maintain fluid and electrolyte balance and delivery of medication. Barium enema is not ordered if perforation is suspected. **Focus:** Prioritization

26. **Ans: 6, 2, 3, 5, 4, 1** Apply a pair of clean gloves before touching the skin. (Note: Visual assessment can be performed without applying gloves; however, the stoma may ooze or require gentle palpation.) The stoma should be assessed for a healthy pink color. Washing, rinsing, drying, and application of a skin barrier help to protect the skin. A good fit prevents gastric contents from spilling onto the skin. **Focus:** Prioritization

Chapter 12: Endocrine Problems, pages 69–72

1. **Ans: 3** Exophthalmos (abnormal protrusion of the eyes) is characteristic of patients with hyperthyroidism due to Graves' disease. Periorbital edema, bradycardia, and hoarse voice are all characteristics of patients with hypothyroidism. **Focus:** Prioritization

2. **Ans: 1** The cardiac problems associated with hyperthyroidism include tachycardia, increased systolic blood pressure, and decreased diastolic blood pressure. Patients with hyperthyroidism also may have increased body temperature related to increased metabolic rate. **Focus:** Delegation/supervision

3. **Ans: 2** Monitoring and recording vital signs are within the educational scope of nursing assistants. An experienced nursing assistant should have been taught how

to monitor the apical pulse. However, the nurse should observe the nursing assistant to be sure that she has mastered this skill. Instructing and teaching patients, as well as performing venipuncture for laboratory samples, are more suited to the educational scope of licensed nurses. In some facilities, an experienced nursing assistant may perform venipuncture, but only after special training. **Focus:** Delegation/supervision, assignment

4. **Ans: 3** Although patients with hypothyroidism often have cardiac problems that include bradycardia, a heart rate of 48/minute may have significant implications for cardiac output and hemodynamic stability. Patients with Graves' disease usually have a rapid heart rate, but 94/minute is within normal limits. The diabetic patient may need sliding scale insulin. This is important but not urgent. Patients with Cushing's disease frequently have dependent edema. **Focus:** Prioritization

5. **Ans: 1** Patients with hypofunction of the adrenal glands often have hypotension and should be instructed to change positions slowly. Once a patient has been instructed, it is appropriate for the nursing assistant to remind the patient of those instructions. Assessing, teaching, and planning nursing care require more education and should be done by licensed nurses. **Focus:** Delegation/supervision

6. **Ans: 4** The presence of crackles in the patient's lungs indicate excess fluid volume due to excess water and sodium reabsorption and may be a symptom of pulmonary edema, which must be treated rapidly. Striae (stretch marks), weight gain, and dependent edema are common findings in patients with Cushing's disease. These findings should be monitored, but are not urgent. **Focus:** Prioritization

7. **Ans: 4** Monitoring vital signs is within the educational scope of the nursing assistant. The nurse should be sure to instruct the nursing assistant that blood pressure measurements are to be done with the cuff on the same arm. Revising the care plan and instructing and assessing patients are beyond the scope of nursing assistants and fall within the purview of licensed nurses. **Focus:** Delegation/supervision

8. **Ans: Palpation of the abdomen** Palpating the abdomen can cause sudden release of catecholamines and severe hypertension. **Focus:** Delegation/supervision

9. **Ans: 1** Rapid weight gain and edema are signs of excessive drug therapy, and the dose of the drug needs to be adjusted. Hypertension, hyperkalemia, and hyperglycemia are common in patients with adrenal hypofunction. **Focus:** Prioritization.

10. **Ans: 1** The presence of glucose in nasal drainage indicates that the fluid is CSF (cerebrospinal fluid) and suggests a CSF leak. Packing is normally inserted in the nares after the surgical incision is closed. Forty to 50 mL per hour is adequate urine output and patients may experience thirst post-operatively. When patients are thirsty, nursing staff should encourage fluid intake. Thirst may be a sign of hypokalemia. The nurse should assess the patient's thirst and check the patient's potassium level. This is not as urgent as the CSF leak. **Focus:** Prioritization

11. **Ans: 2** The 83-year-old patient has no complicating factors at the moment. Providing care for stable and uncomplicated patients is within the LPN's educational preparation and scope of practice, with the care always being provided under the supervision and direction of the RN. The RN should assess the newly post-operative patient and the new admission. The patient who is preparing for discharge after MI may need some complex teaching. **Focus:** Delegation/supervision, assignment

12. **Ans: 1** The parathyroid glands are located on the back of the thyroid gland. The parathyroids are important in maintaining calcium and phosphorus balance. The nurse should be attentive to all patient laboratory values, but calcium and phosphorus are important to monitor after thyroidectomy. **Focus:** Prioritization

13. **Ans: 3** The higher the blood glucose level is over time, the more elevated the glycosylated hemoglobin becomes. Glycosylated hemoglobin is a good indicator of average blood glucose level over the previous 120 days. Fasting glucose and oral glucose tolerance tests are important diagnostic tests. Fingerstick blood glucose monitoring provides information that allows for adjustment of patients' therapeutic regimen. **Focus:** Prioritization

14. **Ans: 4** The nursing assistant's role includes reminding patients about interventions that are already part of the plan of care. Arranging for a diet consult is appropriate to delegate to the unit clerk. Teaching and assessing require additional education and should be completed by licensed nurses. **Focus:** Delegation/supervision, assignment

15. **Ans: 1, 2, 5** Sensory alterations are the major cause of foot complications in diabetic patients, and patients should be taught to examine their feet on a daily basis. Properly fitted shoes protect the patient from foot complications. Broken skin increases the risk of infection. Cotton socks are recommended to absorb moisture. Patients, family, or health care providers may trim toenails. **Focus:** Prioritization

16. **Ans: 3** Profuse perspiration is a symptom of hypoglycemia, a complication of diabetes that needs urgent treatment. A glucose level of 185 will need coverage with sliding-scale insulin, but this is not urgent. Numbness, tingling, and bunions are related to the chronic nature of diabetes and are not urgent. **Focus:** Prioritization

17. **Ans: 1** Checking the bath water temperature is part of assisting with activities of daily living and is within the educational scope of the nursing assistant. Discussion of community resources and teaching and assessing require a higher level of education and are appropriate to the scope of practice of licensed nurses. **Focus:** Delegation

18. **Ans: 2** The new nurse is still orienting to the unit. Appropriate patient assignments at this time include those who are stable and not complex. **Focus:** Assignment

19. **Ans: 2** Rapid, deep respirations (Kussmaul) are symptomatic of DKA. Hammertoe, as well as numbness and tingling, are chronic complications associated with diabetes. Decreased sensitivity and swelling (lipohypertrophy) occur at a site of repeated insulin injections, and treatment involves teaching the patient to rotate injection sites. **Focus:** Prioritization

20. **Ans: 1** The nurse should not leave the patient. The scope of the unit clerk's job includes calling and paging physicians. LPN/LVNs generally do not administer IV push medication. IV fluid administration is not within the scope of nursing assistants. Patients with DKA already have a high glucose level and do not need orange juice. **Focus:** Delegation/supervision

21. **Ans: 2** The signs and symptoms the patient is exhibiting are consistent with hyperglycemia. The RN should

not give the patient additional glucose. All of the other interventions are appropriate for this patient. The RN should also notify the physician at this time. **Focus:** Prioritization

22. **Ans: 4**   The patient with permanent DI requires life-long vasopressin therapy. All of the other statements are appropriate to the home care of this patient. **Focus:** Prioritization

Chapter 13: Integumentary Problems, pages 73–76

1. **Ans: 1**   An LPN/LVN who was experienced in working with post-operative clients would know how to reinforce a dressing. In addition, the LPN/LVN would know to notify the supervising RN about the bleeding. Client teaching and assessments are skills that require more education and a greater scope of practice and are appropriate for registered nurses. **Focus:** Delegation

2. **Ans: 4**   LPN/LVN education and scope of practice include assessment and documentation of common health problems. Choice of the type of dressing to use and assessment for risk factors are more complex skills that are more appropriate to the RN level of practice. LPN/LVNs do function as wound care nurses in some long-term-care facilities, but the choice of dressing type would fall within the RN's role. For a stage 3 ulcer, a nurse with an RN-level education would be most appropriate to select the dressing. Assisting the client to change position is a task included in the nursing assistant's education and would be more appropriate to assign to NA-level staff members. **Focus:** Delegation

3. **Ans: 2**   Facial burns are frequently associated with airway inflammation and swelling, so this client requires the most immediate assessment. The other clients also require rapid assessment or interventions, but not as urgently as the client with facial burns. **Focus:** Prioritization

4. **Ans: 3, 4, 2, 1**   Pain medication should be administered prior to dressing changes, since dressing changes for partial-thickness burns are painful, especially if the dressing change involves removal of eschar. The wound should be debrided prior to obtaining wound cultures to avoid obtaining bacteria that are skin contaminants rather than causes of the wound infection. The antibacterial cream should be applied to the area after debridement to gain the maximum effect. **Focus:** Prioritization

5. **Ans: 3**   A nurse from the oncology unit would be familiar with dressing changes and sterile technique. The charge RN from the burn unit would work closely with the float RN to provide partners to assist in providing care and to answer any questions. Admission assessment and development of the initial care plan, discharge teaching, and splint positioning in burn clients all require expertise in caring for clients with burns. These clients should be assigned to RNs who regularly work on the burn unit. **Focus:** Assignment

6. **Ans: 4**   Irregular borders and a black or variegated color are characteristics associated with malignancy. Striae and toenail thickening or yellowing are common in elderly individuals. Silver-colored scaling is associated with psoriasis, which may need treatment, but is not as urgent a concern as the appearance of the mole. **Focus:** Prioritization

7. **Ans: 1**   A blue color or cyanosis may indicate that the client has significant problems with circulation or ventilation. More detailed assessments are needed immediately. The other data may also indicate health problems in major body systems, but potential respiratory or circulatory abnormalities are the priority. **Focus:** Prioritization

8. **Ans: 1**   Because isotretinoin is associated with a high incidence of birth defects, it is important that the client stop using the medication at least a month before attempting to become pregnant. Nausea and poor night vision are possible adverse effects of isotretinoin, which would require further assessment, but are not as urgent as discussing the fetal risks associated with this medication. The client's concern about whether treatment is effective should be addressed, but this is a lower priority intervention. **Focus:** Prioritization

9. **Ans: 3**   Scheduling the client for an appointment is within the legal scope of practice and training for the medical assistant role. Client teaching, assessment for positive skin reactions to the test, and monitoring for serious allergic reactions are appropriate to the education and practice role of licensed nursing staff. **Focus:** Delegation

10. **Ans: 1**   Systemic use of tetracycline is associated with severe photosensitivity reactions to ultraviolet light. All individuals should be taught about the potential risks associated with overexposure to sunlight or other ultraviolet light, but the client taking tetracycline is at the most immediate risk for severe adverse effects. **Focus:** Prioritization

11. **Ans: 3**   While it is not appropriate for the nursing assistant to plan or implement initial client or family teaching, reinforcement of previous teaching is an important function of the nursing assistant (who is likely to be in the home on a daily basis). Client/family teaching, nutritional assessment and planning, and evaluation for improvement are included in the RN scope of practice. **Focus:** Delegation

12. **Ans: 1**   Medication administration is included in LPN education and scope of practice. Bathing and cleaning clients requires minimal education and would be better delegated to a nursing assistant. Assessment and evaluation of outcomes of care are more complex skills best performed by registered nurses. **Focus:** Delegation

13. **Ans: 2**   The highest priority diagnoses for this client are Acute Pain and Impaired Nutrition. The Acute Pain diagnosis takes precedence because the client's acute oral pain will need to be controlled to improve the ability to eat and to improve nutrition. The assessment data do not indicate that the client's lack of understanding about how the virus is contracted contributed to the infection. (The most frequent cause of oral herpes infection in immunocompromised clients is reactivation of previously acquired herpes simplex.) Disturbed body image is a major concern for the client, but is not as high a priority as the need for pain control and improved nutrition. **Focus:** Prioritization

14. **Ans: 4**   Wheals are frequently associated with allergic reactions, so asking about exposure to new medications is the most appropriate question for this client. The other questions would be useful in assessing the skin health history, but do not directly relate to the client's symptoms. **Focus:** Prioritization

15. **Ans: 2**   With chemical injuries, it is important to remove the chemical from contact with the skin to prevent ongoing damage. The other actions also should be accomplished rapidly; however, rinsing the chemical off is the priority for this client. **Focus:** Prioritization

16. **Ans: 3**   This client's vital signs indicate that the life-threatening complications of sepsis and septic shock may be developing. The other clients also need rapid assessments and/or nursing interventions, but their symptoms do not indicate that they need care as urgently as the febrile and hypotensive client. **Focus:** Prioritization

17. **Ans: 4**   Because aspirin affects platelet aggregation, the client is at increased risk for post-procedure bleeding, and the surgeon will likely reschedule the procedure. The other information is also pertinent, but will not affect the scheduling of the procedure. **Focus:** Prioritization

18. **Ans: 3**   A new graduate would be familiar with the procedure for a sterile dressing change, especially after working for 3 weeks on the unit. Clients who require more complex skills such as admission assessments, pre-procedure teaching, and discharge teaching should be assigned to more experienced RN staff members. **Focus:** Assignment

19. **Ans: 3**   Epigastric pain may indicate that the client is developing peptic ulcers, which require collaborative interventions such as the use of antacids, H$_2$ receptor blockers (e.g., famotidine [Pepcid]), or proton pump inhibitors (e.g., esomeprazole [Nexium]). The elevation in blood glucose, increased appetite, and slight elevation in blood pressure may be related to prednisone use, but are not clinically significant when steroids are used for limited periods and do not require treatment. **Focus:** Prioritization

20. **Ans: 2**   Dairy products inhibit the absorption of tetracycline, so this action would decrease the effectiveness of the antibiotic. The other activities are not appropriate, but would not cause as much potential harm as the administration of tetracycline with milk. Anerobic bacteria would not be likely to grow in a superficial wound. Debridement of burns should be performed by more experienced nursing staff. Pressure garments may be used after graft wounds heal and during the rehabilitation period after a burn injury, but this should be discussed with the client who is ready for rehabilitation, not when the client is admitted. **Focus:** Prioritization

Chapter 14: Renal and Urinary Problems, pages 77–81

1. **Ans: 4**   Providing the equipment that the patient needs to collect the urine sample is within the scope of practice for a nursing assistant. Teaching, planning, and assessing all require additional education and skill, which is appropriate to the scope of practice for professional nurses. **Focus:** Delegation/supervision

2. **Ans: 3**   The presence of 100,000 bacterial colonies/mL in urine or the presence of many WBCs and RBCs indicates a urinary tract infection. The WBC count is within normal limits, and the hematocrit is a little low, which may need follow-up. Neither of these results indicates infection. **Focus:** Prioritization

3. **Ans: 1**   The patient with cystitis who is taking oral antibiotics is stable and has predictable outcomes, therefore appropriate to the scope of practice for the LPN/LVN under the supervision of an RN. The patient with the new order for lithotripsy will need teaching about the procedure, which should be accomplished by the RN. The patient in need of bladder training will need the RN to plan this intervention. The patient with flank pain needs careful and skilled assessment by the RN. **Focus:** Assignment

4. **Ans: 2**   Prostate disease increases the risk of urinary tract infections in men. The patient's wife's UTI should not affect the patient. The catheter usage and kidney stone timeframes are too distant to cause this UTI. **Focus:** Prioritization

5. **Ans: 4**   A cystoscopy is needed to accurately diagnose interstitial cystitis. Urinalysis may show WBCs and RBCs, but no bacteria. The patient will probably need an admission urinalysis, but not daily samples. Intake and output may be assessed, but will not contribute to the diagnosis. Cystitis does not usually affect urine electrolyte levels. **Focus:** Prioritization

6. **Ans: 3**   For uncomplicated cystitis, a 3-day course of antibiotics is an effective treatment, and research has shown that patients are more compliant with shorter antibiotic courses. Seven-day courses of antibiotics are appropriate for complicated cystitis, and 10–14 day courses are prescribed for uncomplicated pyelonephritis. This patient is being discharged and should not be at risk for a nosocomial infection. **Focus:** Prioritization, supervision

7. **Ans: 4**   Women should avoid irritating substances such as bubble bath, nylon underwear, and scented toilet tissue to prevent urinary tract infections. Adequate fluid intake, cranberry juice, and regular voiding are all good strategies for preventing urinary tract infections. **Focus:** Delegation/supervision, prioritization

8. **Ans: 3**   As long as they are alert, aware, and able to resist the urge to urinate, patients with urge incontinence can be taught to control their bladder by starting a schedule for voiding, then increasing the intervals between voids. Patients with functional incontinence related to mental status changes or loss of cognitive function will not be able to follow the bladder-training program. The patient with stress incontinence is better treated with exercises such as pelvic floor (Kegel) exercises to strengthen the pelvic floor muscles. **Focus:** Prioritization

9. **Ans: 1**   Oxybutynin chloride (Ditropan) is an anticholinergic agent, which often causes an extremely dry mouth. The maximum dose is 20 mg per day. This drug can cause tachycardia as a side effect, but does not cause bradycardia. Oxybutynin chloride should be taken between meals because food interferes with absorption of the drug. **Focus:** Prioritization

10. **Ans: 4**   Teaching about bladder emptying, self-catheterization, and medications requires additional knowledge and training and are appropriate to the scope of practice of the RN. The LPN can reinforce information that has already been taught to the patient. **Focus:** Delegation/supervision

11. **Ans: 1**   When patients with urolithiasis pass stones, the stones can cause excruciating pain for up to 24–36 hours. All of the other nursing diagnoses for this patient are accurate; however, at this time, pain is the urgent concern for the patient. **Focus:** Prioritization

12. **Ans: 3**   Bruising is to be expected after lithotripsy. It may be quite extensive and take several weeks to resolve. All of the other statements are accurate for the patient after lithotripsy. **Focus:** Prioritization

13. **Ans: 3, 4**   Both patients will need frequent assessments and medications. The patient on chemotherapy and the newly post-operative patient should not be exposed to any infection. **Focus:** Assignment

14. **Ans: 4**   Administering oral medications appropriately is part of the educational program for the LPN/LVN and is within their scope of practice. Teaching and assessing the patient require additional education and skill and are appropriate to the scope of practice for the RN. **Focus:** Delegation/supervision

15. **Ans: 1, 5, 3, 2, 7, 4, 6, 8**   Before checking post-void residual, you should ask the patient to void and then position him. Next you open the kit and put on sterile gloves, position the patient's penis, clean the meatus, then lubricate and insert the catheter. It is necessary to drain all urine from the bladder to assess the amount of post-void residual the patient has. Finally, the catheter is removed, the penis cleaned, and the urine measured. **Focus:** Prioritization

16. **Ans: 1**   The underlying pathophysiology of nephrotic syndrome involves increased glomerular permeability that allows larger molecules to pass through the membrane into the urine and be removed from the blood. This process causes massive loss of protein, edema formation, and decreased serum albumen levels. Key features include hypertension and renal insufficiency (decreased urine output). Flank pain is seen in patients with acute pyelonephritis. **Focus:** Prioritization

17. **Ans: 2**   Chemotherapy has limited effectiveness against renal cell carcinoma. This form of cancer is usually treated surgically by nephrectomy. **Focus:** Supervision, prioritization

18. **Ans: 1, 2, 3, 5**   A patient with only one kidney should avoid all contact sports and high-risk activities to protect the remaining kidney from injury and preserve renal function. Protective clothing is not adequate to ensure safety. All of the other points are key to preventing renal trauma. **Focus:** Prioritization

19. **Ans: 1, 2, 4, 6**   Administration of oral medications is appropriate to the scope of practice of the LPN/LVN or RN. Assessment of breath sounds requires additional education and skill development and is most appropriate within the scope of practice of the RN, but may be part of an experienced and competent LPN/LVN's observations. All other actions are within the educational preparation and scope of practice for the nursing assistant. **Focus:** Delegation/supervision

20. **Ans: 1**   During the oliguric phase of acute renal failure, patients' urine output is greatly reduced. Fluid boluses and diuretics do not work well. This phase usually lasts from 8 to 15 days. Although there are frequently omissions with regard to recording intake and output, this is probably not the cause of the patient's decreased urine output. Retention of sodium and water is the rationale for giving furosemide, not the reason that it is ineffective. Nitrogenous wastes build up as a result of the kidneys' inability to perform their elimination function. **Focus:** Delegation/supervision

21. **Ans: 2**   A nurse from SICU is thoroughly familiar with the care of newly post-operative patients. The patient scheduled for lithotripsy may need education about the procedure. The newly admitted patient needs an in-depth admission assessment, and the patient with chronic renal failure needs teaching about peritoneal dialysis. All of these interventions/actions would best be accomplished by an experienced nurse with expertise in the care of patients with renal problems. **Focus:** Assignment

22. **Ans: 1**   Gentamicin can be a highly nephrotoxic substance. Creatinine and BUN should be monitored for elevations indicating possible nephrotoxicity. All of the other measures are important, but are not specific to gentamicin therapy. **Focus:** Prioritization

23. **Ans: 2**   Patients with acute renal failure usually go though a diuretic phase 2–6 weeks after the onset of the oliguric phase. The diuresis can result in an output of up to 10 L/day of dilute urine. During this phase, it is important to monitor for electrolyte and fluid imbalances. This is followed by the recovery phase. A patient with ARF due to hypovolemia would receive IV fluids to correct the problem; however, this would not necessarily cause the onset of diuresis. **Focus:** Supervision

24. **Ans: 1**   CVVH is a continuous renal replacement therapy that is prescribed for patients with renal failure who are critically ill and do not tolerate the rapid shifts in fluids and electrolytes that are associated with hemodialysis. A teaching plan is not urgent at this time. Continuous veno-venous therapy does not require a specific mean arterial pressure and utilizes a blood pump to propel blood through the blood tubing circuit. When a patient urgently needs a procedure, morning care does not take priority and may be deferred until later in the day. **Focus:** Prioritization

Chapter 15: Reproductive Problems, pages 83–87

1. **Ans: 3**   A palpable bladder and restlessness are indicators of bladder distention, which would require action (such as insertion of a catheter) in order to empty the bladder. The other data would be consistent with the client's diagnosis of BPH. More detailed assessment may be indicated, but no immediate action is needed. **Focus:** Prioritization

2. **Ans: 4**   Irregularly shaped and nontender lumps are consistent with a diagnosis of breast cancer, so this client needs immediate referral for diagnostic tests such as mammography or ultrasound. The other information is not unusual and does not indicate the need for immediate action. **Focus:** Prioritization

3. **Ans: 1**   An LPN/LVN working in a PACU would be expected to check dressings for bleeding and alert RN staff members if bleeding occurred. The other tasks are more appropriate for nursing staff with RN level education and licensure. **Focus:** Delegation

4. **Ans: 2**   Positioning the client's arm is a task that a nursing assistant who works on a surgical unit would be educated to do. Client teaching and assessment are RN-level skills. Elastic bandages are not usually used in the immediate post-operative period because they inhibit collateral lymphatic drainage. **Focus:** Delegation

5. **Ans: 4**   The bladder spasms may indicate that blood clots are obstructing the catheter, which would indicate the need for irrigation of the catheter with 30–50 mL of saline using a piston syringe. The other data would all be normal after a TURP, but the client may need some teaching about the usual post-TURP symptoms and care. **Focus:** Prioritization

6. **Ans: 4**   Because tamsulosin blocks alpha-receptors in the peripheral arterial system, the most significant side effects are orthostatic hypotension and dizziness. To avoid falls, it is important that the client change position slowly. The other information is also accurate and may be included in client teaching, but is not as important as decreasing the risk for falls. **Focus:** Prioritization

7. **Ans: 2** Hemorrhage is a major complication after TURP and should be reported to the surgeon immediately. The other assessment data also indicate a need for nursing action, but not as urgently. **Focus:** Prioritization

8. **Ans: 1** Reinforcement of previous teaching is an expected role of the LPN. Planning/implementing client initial teaching and documentation of a client's discharge assessment should be accomplished by experienced RN staff members. **Focus:** Delegation

9. **Ans: 4** It is important to assess oxygenation because the client's shortness of breath may indicate a pulmonary embolus, a serious complication of TURP. Dorsiflexion of the foot should not be done if a deep vein thrombosis is suspected, since this may dislodge thrombus. The other activities are appropriate, but are not as high a priority as ensuring that oxygenation is adequate. **Focus:** Prioritization

10. **Ans: 1** This client has symptoms of testicular torsion, an emergency which needs immediate assessment and intervention, since it can lead to testicular ischemia and necrosis within a few hours. The other clients also have symptoms of acute problems (primary syphilis, acute bacterial prostatitis, and prostatic hypertrophy and urinary retention), which also need rapid assessment and intervention. **Focus:** Prioritization

11. **Ans: 2, 1, 3, 4** Bladder spasms are usually caused by the presence of clots obstructing the catheter, so irrigation should be the first action taken. Administration of analgesics may help to reduce spasm. Administration of a bolus of IV fluids is commonly used in the immediate post-operative period to help maintain fluid intake and increase urinary flow. Oral fluid intake should be encouraged once you are sure that the client is not nauseated and has adequate bowel tones. **Focus:** Prioritization

12. **Ans: 3** Sildenafil is a potent vasodilator and has caused cardiac arrest in clients who were also taking nitrates such as nitroglycerin. The other client data indicate the need for further assessment and/or teaching, but it is essential for the client who uses nitrates to avoid concurrent use of sildenafil. **Focus:** Prioritization

13. **Ans: 2** Administration of narcotics and the associated client monitoring are included in LPN education and scope of practice. Assessments and teaching are more complex skills that require RN-level education and will be best accomplished by an RN with experience caring for clients with this diagnosis. **Focus:** Delegation

14. **Ans: 3** Safe ambulation of clients is included in nursing assistant education, and an experienced nursing assistant would be expected to accomplish this task. The other clients will need assessments and/or teaching by an RN. **Focus:** Assignment

15. **Ans: 4, 3, 2, 1** The bilateral orchiectomy client needs immediate assessment, since confusion may be an indicator of serious post-operative complications such as hemorrhage, infection, or pulmonary embolism. The client who had a perineal prostatectomy should be assessed next, since pain medication may be needed to allow him to perform essential post-operative activities such as deep breathing, coughing, and ambulating. The vaginal hysterectomy client's anxiety needs further assessment next. Although the breast implant client has questions about care of the drains at the surgical site, there is nothing in the report indicating that these need to be addressed immediately. **Focus:** Prioritization

16. **Ans: 3** Although sepsis is a rare complication of transrectal prostate biopsy, it is important that the client receive teaching about checking his temperature and calling the physician for any fever or other signs of systemic infection. It is important that the client understand that the test results will not be available immediately, but that he will be notified about the results. Transient rectal bleeding may occur after the biopsy, but bleeding that lasts for more than a few hours indicates that there may have been rectal trauma. **Focus:** Prioritization

17. **Ans: 4** Cramping or aching abdominal pain is common after D&C; however, sharp, continuous pain may indicate uterine perforation, which would require immediate notification of the physician. The other data indicate a need for ongoing assessment or interventions. Transient blood pressure elevation may occur due to the stress response after surgery. Bleeding following the procedure is expected, but should decrease over the first 2 hours. And while the oxygen saturation is not at an unsafe level, interventions to improve the saturation should be accomplished. **Focus:** Prioritization

18. **Ans: 2, 4, 5** Assisting with catheter care, ambulation, and hygiene is included in home health aide education and would be expected activities for this staff member. Client assessment and teaching are the responsibility of RN members of the home health team. **Focus:** Delegation

19. **Ans: 1** Because the most likely source of the bacteria causing the TSS is the client's tampon, it is essential to remove it first. The other actions should be implemented in the following order: administer oxygen (essential to maximize O_2 delivery to tissues), obtain blood cultures (best obtained prior to initiating antibiotic therapy to obtain accurate culture and susceptibility results), and infuse nafcillin (rapid initiation of antibiotic therapy will decrease bacterial release of toxins). **Focus:** Prioritization

20. **Ans: 2** Right calf swelling indicates the possible presence of deep vein thrombosis. This will change the plan of care, since the client should be placed on bedrest, while the usual plan is to ambulate the client as soon as possible after surgery. The other data indicate the need for common post-operative nursing actions such as having the client cough, assessing her pain, and increasing her fluid intake. **Focus:** Prioritization

21. **Ans: 3** Clients with intracavitary implants are kept in bed during the treatment to avoid dislodgement of the implant. The other actions may also require you to intervene by providing guidance to the student. Minimal time should be spent close to clients who are receiving internal radiation, asking the client about her reaction to losing child-bearing abilities may be inappropriate at this time, and clients are frequently placed on low-residue diets to decrease bowel distention while implants are in place. **Focus:** Prioritization

22. **Ans: 1** The client has symptoms of a urinary tract infection. Inserting a straight catheter will enable you to obtain an uncontaminated urine specimen for culture and susceptibility testing before the antibiotic is started. In addition, the client is probably not emptying her bladder fully because of the painful urination. The antibiotic should be initiated as rapidly as possible once the urine specimen is obtained. Administration

of acetaminophen is the lowest priority, because the client's temperature is not dangerously elevated. **Focus:** Prioritization

23. **Ans: 2** After an A and P repair, it is essential that the bladder be empty to avoid putting pressure on the suture lines. The abdominal firmness and tenderness indicate that the client's bladder is distended. The physician should be notified and an order for catheterization obtained. The other data also indicate a need for further assessment of her cardiac status and actions such as having the client cough and deep breathe, but are not such immediate concerns. **Focus:** Prioritization

24. **Ans: 3** The client should be positioned in a semi-Fowler's position to minimize the risk of abscess development higher in the abdomen. The other actions also require correction, but not as rapidly. Tampon use is not contraindicated after an episode of PID, although some sources recommend not using tampons during the acute infection. Heat application to the abdomen and pelvis is used for pain relief. Intercourse is safe a few weeks after effective treatment for PID. **Focus:** Prioritization

25. **Ans: 2** "Red man syndrome" occurs when vancomycin is infused too quickly. Because the client needs the medication to treat PID, the vancomycin should not be discontinued. Antihistamines may help decrease the flushing, but vancomycin should be administered over at least 60 minutes. **Focus:** Prioritization

26. **Ans: 4** Wound dehiscence or evisceration may cause shock, so the first action should be to assess the client's blood pressure and heart rate. The next action should be to ensure that the abdominal contents remain moist by covering the wound and loops of intestine with dressings soaked with sterile normal saline. The physician should be notified. The nurse should not attempt to replace any eviscerated organs back into the abdominal cavity. **Focus:** Prioritization

27. **Ans: 3** LPN/LVN education includes vital sign monitoring; an experienced LPN/LVN would also know to report changes in vital signs to the RN. The paracentesis tray could be obtained by a nursing assistant or unit clerk. Client admission assessment and teaching require RN-level education and experience, although part of the data gathering may be done by the LPN/LVN. **Focus:** Delegation

Chapter 16: Medical-Surgical Emergencies, pages 89—94

1. **Ans: 3** Triage requires at least one experienced RN. Pairing an experienced RN with inexperienced RN provides opportunities for mentoring. Advanced practice nurses are qualified to perform triage; however, their services are usually required in other areas of the ED. An LPN/LVN is not qualified to perform the initial patient assessment or decision making. Pairing an experienced RN with a nursing assistant is the second best option, because the assistant can obtain vital signs and assist in transporting. **Focus:** Assignment

2. **Ans: 2, 1, 4, 3** An irritable infant with fever and petechiae should be further assessed for other meningeal signs. The patient with the head wound needs additional history and assessment for intracranial pressure. The patient with moderate abdominal pain is uncomfortable, but not unstable at this point. For the ankle injury, medical evaluation can be delayed 24–48 hours if necessary. **Focus:** Prioritization

3. **Ans: 3** A brief neurologic assessment to determine level of consciousness and pupil reaction is part of the primary survey. Vital signs, assessment of the abdomen, and initiation of pulse oximetry are considered part of the secondary survey. **Focus:** Prioritization

4. **Ans: 4** Chest pain is considered an emergent priority, which is defined as potentially life-threatening. Patients with urgent priority need treatment within 2 hours of triage (e.g., kidney stones). Non-urgent conditions can wait for hours or even days. (High urgent is not commonly used; however, in 5-tier triage systems, High urgent patients fall between Emergent and Urgent in terms of the time lapsing prior to treatment.) **Focus:** Prioritization

5. **Ans: 1** The nursing assistant can assist with the removal of outer clothing, which allows the heat to dissipate from the child's skin. Advising and explaining are teaching functions that are the responsibility of the RN. Tepid baths are not usually performed because of potential for rebound and shivering. **Focus:** Delegation

6. **Ans: 4** The homeless person has symptoms of heat stroke, a medical emergency, which increases risk for brain damage. Elderly patients are at risk for heat syncope and should be educated to rest in a cool area and avoid future similar situations. The runner is having heat cramps, which can be managed with rest and fluids. The housewife is experiencing heat exhaustion, and management includes fluids (IV or parenteral) and cooling measures. The prognosis for recovery is good. **Focus:** Prioritization

7. **Ans: 2, 4, 1, 3, 5** Establish unresponsiveness first. (The patient may have fallen and sustained a minor injury.) If the patient is unresponsive, get help and have someone initiate the code. Performing the chin lift or jaw thrust maneuver opens the airway. The nurse is then responsible for starting CPR. CPR should not be interrupted until the patient recovers or it is determined that heroic efforts have been exhausted. A crash cart should be at the site when the code team arrives; however, basic CPR can be effectively performed until the team arrives. **Focus:** Prioritization

8. **Ans: 1** Nursing assistants are trained in basic cardiac life support and can perform chest compressions. The use of the bag-valve mask requires practice and usually a respiratory therapist will perform this function. The nurse or the respiratory therapist should provide PRN assistance during intubation. The defibrillator pads are clearly marked; however, placement should be done by the RN or physician because of the potential for skin damage and electrical arcing. **Focus:** Delegation

9. **Ans: 3** The patient is hyperventilating secondary to anxiety, and breathing into a paper bag will allow rebreathing of carbon dioxide. Also, encouraging slow breathing will help. Other treatments such as oxygen and medication may be needed if other causes are identified. **Focus:** Prioritization

10. **Ans: 3** The fast track clinic will deal with relatively stable patients. Triage, trauma, and pediatric medicine should be staffed with experienced nurses who know the hospital routines and policies and can rapidly locate equipment. **Focus:** Assignment

11. **Ans: 1** Iron is a toxic substance that can lead to massive hemorrhage, coma, shock, and hepatic failure. Deferoxamine is an antidote that can be used for severe cases of iron poisoning. Other information needs additional investigation, but will not change the immediate

diagnostic testing or treatment plan. **Focus:** Prioritization

12. **Ans: 3**   The LPN/LVN is able to listen and provide emotional support for her patients. The other tasks are the responsibility of an RN or, if available, a SANE (sexual assault nurse examiner) who has received training to assess, collect and safeguard evidence, and care for these victims. **Focus:** Delegation

13. **Ans: 3, 2, 4, 1**   The victim should be removed from the cold environment first, then the rewarming process can be initiated. It will be painful, so give pain medication prior to immersing the feet in warmed water. **Focus:** Prioritization

14. **Ans: 3**   The only correct intervention is 3. The digits should be gently cleansed with normal saline, wrapped in sterile gauze moistened with saline, and placed in a plastic bag or container. The container is then placed on ice. **Focus:** Delegation

15. **Ans: 2**   IV lorazepam (Ativan) is the drug of choice for status epilepticus. Tegretol is used in the management of generalized tonic-clonic, absence or mixed type seizures, but it does not come in an IV form. PO (per os) medications are inappropriate for this emergency situation. Magnesium sulfate is given to control seizures in toxemia of pregnancy. **Focus:** Prioritization

16. **Ans: 3**   Parent refusal is an absolute contraindication; therefore, the physician must be notified. Tetanus status can be addressed later. The RN can restart the IV and provide information about conscious sedation; if the parent is still not satisfied, the physician can give more information. **Focus:** Prioritization

17. **Ans: 4**   The patient presents with symptoms of alcohol abuse and there is a risk for Wernicke's syndrome, which is caused by a thiamine deficiency. Multiple drug abuse is not uncommon; however, there is nothing in the question that suggests an opiate overdose that requires naloxone. Additional information or the results of the blood alcohol level are part of the total treatment plan but should not delay the immediate treatment. **Focus:** Prioritization

18. **Ans: 3**   Postmortem care requires some turning, cleaning, lifting, etc., and the nursing assistant is able to assist with these duties. The RN should take responsibility for the other tasks to help the family begin the grieving process. In cases of questionable death, belongings may be retained for evidence, so the chain of custody would have to be maintained. **Focus:** Delegation

19. **Ans: 3, 4, 2, 1**   Auscultating and confirming equal bilateral breath sounds should be performed in rapid succession. If the sounds are not equal or if the sounds are heard over the mid-epigastric area, tube placement must be corrected immediately. Securing the tube is appropriate while waiting for the x-ray study. **Focus:** Prioritization

20. **Ans: 2**   An impaled object may be providing a tamponade effect, and removal can precipitate sudden hemodynamic decompensation. Additional history including a more definitive description of the blood loss, depth of penetration, and medical history should be obtained. Other information, such as the dirt on the stick or history of diabetes, is important in the overall treatment plan, but can be addressed later. **Focus:** Prioritization

21. **Ans: 1**   The patient demonstrates neurologic hyperreactivity and is on the verge of a seizure. Patient safety

is the priority. The patient needs chlordiazepoxide (Librium) to decrease neurologic irritability and phenytoin (Dilantin) for seizures. Thiamine and haloperidol (Haldol) will also be ordered to address the other problems. The other diagnoses are pertinent but not as immediate. **Focus:** Prioritization

22. **Ans: 2**   The stinger will continue to release venom into the skin, so prompt removal of the stinger is advised. Cool compresses and antihistamines can follow. The caller should be further advised about symptoms that require 911 assistance. **Focus:** Prioritization

23. **Ans: 4**   The asymptomatic patient is currently stable but should be observed for delayed pulmonary edema, cerebral edema, or pneumonia. Teaching and care of critical patients is an RN responsibility. Removing clothing can be delegated to a nursing assistant. **Focus:** Delegation

24. **Ans: 1**   Cats' mouths contain a virulent organism, *Pasteurella multocida*, that can lead to septic arthritis or bacteremia. There is also a risk for tendon damage due to deep puncture wounds. These wounds are usually not sutured. A tetanus shot can be given before discharge. **Focus:** Prioritization

25. **Ans: 4, 2, 3, 1**   The patient with a pulsating mass has an abdominal aneurysm that may rupture and he may decompensate suddenly. The 11-year-old boy needs evaluation to rule out appendicitis. The woman needs evaluation for gallbladder problems that appear to be worsening. The 35-year-old man has food poisoning, which is usually self-limiting. **Focus:** Prioritization

26. **Ans: 4**   At least one representative from each group should be included because all employees are potential targets for violence in the ED. **Focus:** Assignment

27. **Ans: 1**   A deviated trachea is a symptom of tension pneumothorax. All of the other symptoms need to be addressed, but are of lesser priority. **Focus:** Prioritization

28. **Ans: 3, 2, 4, 1, 5, 6, 7**   For a multiple trauma victim, many interventions will occur simultaneously as team members assist in the resuscitation. Methods to open the airway such as the chin lift or jaw thrust can be used simultaneously while assessing for spontaneous respirations. However, airway and oxygenation are priority. Starting IVs for fluid resuscitation is part of supporting circulation. (EMS will usually establish at least one IV in the field.) Nursing assistants can be directed to take vitals and remove clothing. Foley catheter is necessary to closely monitor output. **Focus:** Prioritization

29. **Ans: 1**   In preparing for disasters, the RN should be aware of the emergency response plan. The plan gives guidance that includes roles of team members, responsibilities, and mechanisms of reporting. Signs and symptoms of many agents will mimic common complaints, such as flu-like symptoms. Discussions with colleagues and supervisors may help the individual nurse to sort through ethical dilemmas related to potential danger to self. **Focus:** Prioritization

30. **Ans: 1**   Safety is a priority for this patient, and she should not return to a place where violence could reoccur. The other options are important for the long-term management of this case. **Focus:** Prioritization

31. **Ans: 3, 4, 2, 5, 1**   The first priority is to protect personnel, unaffected patients, bystanders, and the facility. PPG should be donned prior to exposure to victims. Decontamination of victims in a separate area is fol-

lowed by triage and treatment. The incident should be reported according to protocol as information about the number of persons involved, history, signs, and symptoms becomes available. **Focus:** Prioritization

PART 3

Case Study 1: Chest Pressure, Indigestion, Nausea, and Vomiting, pages 97–99

1. **Ans: 4**   Monitoring and recording intake and output are within the scope of practice for a nursing assistant. Placing the client on telemetry, venipuncture, and obtaining ECGs require additional education and training. Placing leads may be done by unlicensed assistive personnel (UAPs) in some facilities along with venipuncture and ECG. However, these UAPs would require additional specialized training. These actions are generally considered to be within the scope of practice of licensed nurses. **Focus:** Delegation

2. **Ans: 3**   Cardiac monitoring is the highest priority because the client's heart rate is rapid and irregular, and the client is experiencing chest pressure. The client is at risk for life-threatening dysrhythmias such as frequent PVCs. Obtaining vital signs every 2 hours and cardiac markers and 12-lead ECG every 6 hours are important, but cardiac monitoring takes precedence for the reasons stated above. **Focus:** Prioritization

3. **Ans: CK-MB**   Myoglobin is the first marker to rise, but it is not specific to myocardial damage. CK-MB is specific and diagnostic for myocardial damage. **Focus:** Knowledge

4. **Ans: 1**   With frequent PVCs, the client is at risk for life-threatening dysrhythmias such as ventricular tachycardia or ventricular fibrillation. Amiodarone is an antidysrhythmic drug used to control ventricular dysrhythmias. Nitroglycerin and morphine can be used for chest pain relief. Atenolol is a beta blocker, which can be used to control heart rate and decrease blood pressure. **Focus:** Prioritization

5. **Ans: 2**   CK and CK-MB are elevated and diagnostic for acute myocardial infarction. Even though all the other laboratory values are abnormal, none of them is life threatening. **Focus:** Prioritization

6. **Ans: 1**   Morphine sulfate has been ordered to relieve the chest discomfort that is common in the setting of acute myocardial infarction. Relief from the chest pain is the highest priority at this time. Ranitidine is an H₂ blocker used to prevent gastric ulcers. Scheduling an echocardiogram or drawing coagulation studies, while important, will not help relieve chest discomfort. **Focus:** Prioritization

7. **Ans: 1, 2, 6**   Vital signs, recording intake and output, and assisting clients with activities of daily living are all within the scope of practice of the nursing assistant. Administration of IV drugs, venipuncture for laboratory tests, and assessment are beyond the scope of practice for nursing assistants. **Focus:** Delegation/supervision, assignment

8. **Ans: 4**   Monitoring and recording vital signs are within the scope of practice of the nursing assistant. When a nursing assistant makes a mistake, it is best to communicate specifically, stressing the importance of recording the vital signs after they have been assessed. Supervision should be done in a supportive rather than confrontational manner. Notification of the nurse manager is not appropriate at this time. Reprimanding the nursing assistant in front of others is not appropriate. **Focus:** Delegation/supervision

9. **Ans: 2**   Chest pain can be an indicator of additional myocardial muscle damage. Additional episodes of chest pain significantly affect the client's plan of care. Small increases in heart rate and blood pressure after activity are to be expected. The temperature elevation should continue to be monitored for any additional elevation. **Focus:** Prioritization, delegation/supervision

10. **Ans: 1**   HCTZ is a thiazide diuretic used to correct edema and lower blood pressure. A side effect of HCTZ is loss of potassium, and clients may require potassium supplements. Captopril is an ACE inhibitor and will lower blood pressure. It is never appropriate to take twice the dose of this drug. **Focus:** Prioritization

Case Study 2: Dyspnea and Shortness of Breath, pages 101–102

1. **Ans: 2**   The patient's major problems, at this time, are focused on airway and breathing. The patient's anxiety is most likely directly related to his breathing difficulty. An acid-base imbalance may result from the patient's breathing problem, but this is not the highest priority at the moment. **Focus:** Prioritization

2. **Ans: 1**   Baseline arterial blood gas results are important in planning the care for this patient. The unit clerk can schedule the pulmonary function tests and chest x-ray. The albuterol is a routine order and should be administered after baseline ABGs are obtained to avoid altering the test results. **Focus:** Prioritization

3. **Ans: 4**   Increasing oxygen flow for a patient based on a physician's order is within the scope of practice for LPN/LVNs. While taking vital signs is also within the scope of practice for LPN/LVNs, this may be more appropriately delegated to a nursing assistant. Arterial laboratory draws are not within the LPN/LVN's scope of practice. Handheld nebulizers are usually administered by respiratory therapists. **Focus:** Delegation/supervision

4. **Ans: 1, 4, 6**   Assisting patients with activities of daily living such as toileting is within the scope of practice of nursing assistants. Once licensed nurses or respiratory therapists have taught the patient to use incentive spirometry, the nursing assistant can play a role in reminding the patient to use it. Nursing assistants can participate in encouraging patients to drink adequate fluids. Assessing and teaching are not within the scope of practice for nursing assistants. Checking pulse oximetry could be appropriate for experienced nursing assistants once they have been taught how to use the pulse oximetry device to gather additional data. **Focus:** Delegation/supervision, assignment

5. **Ans: 3**   Barrel chest and clubbed fingers are signs of chronic COPD. The patient had a productive cough on admission to the hospital. Bilateral crackles are a new finding and indicate fluid-filled alveoli and pulmonary edema. Fluid in the alveoli affects gas exchange and can result in worsening arterial blood gas results. **Focus:** Prioritization

6. **Ans: 1**   Furosemide (Lasix) is a loop diuretic. The uses of this drug include treatment of pulmonary edema. Intake and output records and daily weights are important in documenting the effectiveness of the medication. A side effect of this drug is hypokalemia, and some patients are also prescribed a potassium supplement when taking this medication. **Focus:** Prioritization

7. **Ans: 3** The patient's temperature was elevated on admission. Further elevation indicates ongoing infection. The physician needs to be notified and an appropriate treatment plan started. All of the other pieces of information are important, but are not urgent. The patient's incontinence is not new. **Focus:** Supervision, prioritization.

8. **Ans: 4** The heart rate and blood pressure are slightly increased from admission and the respiratory rate is slightly decreased. The continued elevation in temperature indicates a probable respiratory tract infection that needs to be recognized and treated. **Focus:** Prioritization

9. **Ans: 2** Discharge planning and administration of IV antibiotics are more appropriate to the scope of practice of the RN. However, in some states LPN/LVNs with special training may administer IV antibiotics. Check the regulations in your state. Administering oral medications is appropriate to delegate to LPN/LVNs. Although the LPN/LVN could weigh the patient, this intervention is appropriate to the scope of practice for nursing assistants. **Focus:** Delegation/supervision

Case Study 3: A Nursing Team Leader Caring for Multiple Clients, pages 103–105

1. **Ans: 1, 3, 4, 6** It is important to recognize that the RN continues to be accountable for *all* client care on this team. Appropriate client assignments include clients whose conditions are stable and not complex. You could assign nursing care tasks for Mr. C., but would need to do the cardiac catheterization teaching. The LPN/LVN could then reinforce your teaching. Ms. J. is currently experiencing chest pain, and Ms. B. is a complex new admission, so neither is suitable for assignment of care to an LPN. **Focus:** Assignment, delegation/supervision

2. **Ans: 2** Although it is important for the nurse to see all of these clients, Ms. J.'s assessment takes priority. Her chest pain may indicate coronary artery blockage and acute heart attack. None of the other clients' needs is life threatening. **Focus:** Prioritization

3. **Ans: 3** Cardiac catheterization is usually accomplished by inserting a large-bore needle into the femoral vein and/or artery. Clients are routinely restricted to bedrest for 6–8 hours after the procedure to prevent hemorrhage. Family members are usually permitted to visit as soon as the client returns to the room. **Focus:** Prioritization

4. **Ans: 4, 1, 2, 1, 2, 1, 2, 1, 4, 3** The ECG should be completed first because the physician has ordered that it be done during episodes of pain. Blood pressure and heart rate should be checked before and after administering nitroglycerin for each of the three doses. Hypotension is a side effect of nitroglycerin. Nitroglycerin is usually tried before giving morphine sulfate. **Focus:** Prioritization

5. **Ans: 4** Assessment and teaching are more appropriate to the educational preparation of licensed nursing staff. The nursing assistant could check pulse oximetry after she has been oriented and taught to use the device. Monitoring and recording intake and output are within the educational scope of nursing assistants. **Focus:** Assignment, delegation/supervision

6. **Ans: 1** A temperature elevation to 102°F is an indicator of an infectious process. The other vital signs are within or close to normal limits. **Focus:** Delegation/supervision

7. **Ans: 3** Acute chest pain can indicate myocardial ischemia, coronary artery blockage, and/or myocardial damage. The nursing assistant's question should be answered with the most accurate response. While the unit may have protocols that the nursing assistant should be familiar with, 4 is not the most accurate response. **Focus:** Prioritization

8. **Ans: 2** Assisting clients with activities of daily living such as feeding is most appropriate to the scope of practice for nursing assistants. **Focus:** Delegation/supervision, assignment

9. **Ans: 3** The nurse should gather more information before notifying the physician. Pulse oximetry assessment provides information about the client's oxygenation status. Clients with COPD are usually kept on low-dose oxygen because their stimulus for breathing is low oxygen levels. Coughing and deep breathing provide the benefit of helping to mobilize secretions and may be encouraged after checking oxygenation level if you detect excessive secretions on assessment (e.g., crackles). **Focus:** Prioritization

10. **Ans: 1** This client's temperature elevation is most likely due to an infection. The physician must be notified to modify the client's plan of care. Administering acetaminophen, if it has been ordered by the physician, and removing extra blankets may decrease the client's temperature, but it will not treat the infection. **Focus:** Prioritization

11. **Ans: Infection of the bladder** The client's temperature elevation indicates an infectious process. For elderly clients with bladder infections, changes in level of consciousness are frequently a sign. **Focus:** Knowledge

12. **Ans: 2** Assisting clients with activities of daily living are appropriate to the educational preparation and scope of practice for nursing assistants. Teaching, assessing, and administering medications fall within the scope of practice of licensed nurses. **Focus:** Delegation/supervision

13. **Ans: 2** A common side effect of beta-adrenergic agonists such as albuterol is increased heart rate. MDIs such as albuterol are commonly prescribed for clients with COPD to use as needed to dilate the airways when experiencing shortness of breath. While the other factors are important and may have contributed to the client's COPD, they may not have contributed to the increase in heart rate. **Focus:** Prioritization

14. **Ans: 4** Standards of practice for the use of restraints require that nurses attempt alternative strategies before requesting a physician's order for a client to be restrained. A physician's order is required for continued use of restraints but can be gotten after the fact if the client's actions may cause self injury. **Focus:** Prioritization, delegation/supervision

15. **Ans: 3** The nursing assistant is new to the unit and may need assistance or instruction regarding the completion of this assignment, although it is within the NA scope of practice. **Focus:** Delegation/supervision, assignment

16. **Ans: Right Task, Right Person, Right Circumstance, Right Direction/Communication, and Right Supervision** According to the National Counsel of State Boards of Nursing, the 5 Rights are essential for the process of delegation. They are: "The Right Task is assigned to the Right Person in the Right Circumstances. The RN then offers the Right Direction/

Communication and Right Supervision. **Focus:** Delegation/supervision, assignment

Case Study 4: Shortness of Breath, Edema, and Decreased Urine Output, pages 107–109

1. **Ans: 2**   All of these findings are important, but only the presence of crackles in both lungs is urgent because it signifies fluid-filled alveoli and interruption of adequate gas exchange and oxygenation, possibly pulmonary edema. The patient's peripheral edema is not new. The faint pulses are most likely due to the presence of peripheral edema. The dry and peeling skin is a result of chronic diabetes that merits careful monitoring to prevent infection. **Focus:** Prioritization

2. **Ans: 3**   Teaching, instructing, and assessing are all functions that require additional education and preparation. These interventions fall within the scope of the professional nurse. Providing the patient with ice for the urine collection, as well as reminding the patient to collect her urine, fit the scope of practice for the nursing assistant. **Focus:** Delegation/supervision

3. **Ans: 1**   A patient with a serum potassium of 7.0–8.0 or higher is at risk for electrocardiographic changes and fatal dysrhythmias. You should notify the physician immediately about this potassium level. While the serum creatinine and blood urea nitrogen are quite high, these levels are commonly reached before patients experience symptoms of CRF. The serum calcium level is low, but not life threatening. Keep in mind that there is an inverse relationship between calcium and phosphorus, so when calcium is low, expect phosphorus to be high. **Focus:** Prioritization

4. **Ans: 4**   Sodium polystyrene sulfonate (Kayexalate) removes potassium from the body by exchanging sodium for potassium in the large intestine. Diuretics such as furosemide do not work well in CRF. The patient may need a calcium supplement for the hypocalcemia and subcutaneous epoetin to treat anemia. **Focus:** Prioritization

5. **Ans: 1**   Insertion of an intermittent catheter is within the scope of practice for the LPN/LVN, although LPN/LVNs must be under the supervision of an RN. Planning care, teaching respiratory care techniques, and discussing options such as renal replacement therapies all generally require additional education and training. In many acute care hospitals, LPN/LVNs auscultate breath sounds as a part of their observations, and RNs follow up with overall assessment and synthesis of data. These interventions are more appropriate to the scope of practice for the RN. **Focus:** Delegation/supervision

6. **Ans: 2**   Checking vital signs usually includes measuring oral body temperature. Because the patient just finished drinking a cup of hot tea, an oral temperature measurement would be inaccurately high. All of the other actions are appropriate and within the scope of practice for a nursing assistant. **Focus:** Delegation/supervision

7. **Ans: 1, 2, 3, 5**   The usual fluid restriction for patients with chronic renal failure is 500–700 mL plus urine output. All of the other actions are appropriate for a patient with fluid overload. **Focus:** Prioritization

8. **Ans: 2**   Even after beginning HD, patients are still required to restrict fluid intake. Additionally, patients on HD have nutritional restrictions (e.g., protein, potassium, phosphorus, and sodium). All of the other patient statements indicate appropriate understanding of teaching about HD. **Focus:** Prioritization

9. **Ans: 3**   Temporary dialysis accesses are only to be used for HD. The supervising nurse should stop the orienting nurse before the temporary HD system is interrupted. Breaking into the system increases the risk for complications such as infection or bleeding. The blood pressure should always be assessed on the non-dialysis arm. Bleeding should always be monitored in postoperative patients. Oxycodone, when ordered by the physician, is an appropriate analgesic for moderate to moderately severe pain. **Focus:** Delegation/supervision

10. **Ans: 3**   Changes in level of consciousness during or after HD can signal dialysis disequilibrium syndrome, a life-threatening situation that requires early recognition and treatment with anticonvulsants. A decrease in weight and blood pressure is to be expected as a result of dialysis therapy. A small amount of drainage on the dressing is common after HD. **Focus:** Prioritization

11. **Ans: 1**   Obtaining vital signs and weighing the patient are all within the educational scope of the nursing assistant. Assessing the patient's access site for bleeding, bruit, and thrill requires additional education and skill that is appropriate to the licensed nurse. Nursing assistants can remind and reinforce instructions given by the nurse, but teaching and instructing are appropriate to the scope of practice for licensed nurses. **Focus:** Delegation/supervision

12. **Ans: 4**   Epogen (erythropoietin alpha) is given two to three times a week to treat anemia. However, it is given either by IV or SC route. Most commonly, Epogen is given subcutaneously. All of the other statements about CRF patient medications are accurate. **Focus:** Delegation/supervision

Case Study 5: Abdominal Pain, Polyuria, Vomiting, and Thirst, pages 111–113

1. **Ans: 1, 2, 5, 6, 7**   Onset of symptoms and the amount of fluid loss help to determine acuity. Pain assessment on the abdomen should be done as a baseline; his pain is probably associated with diabetic ketoacidosis (DKA), but infection or trauma could also be factors. If Mr. D. had insulin today, it will affect the emergency insulin therapy that the physician will order. Information about allergies should be obtained on all clients regardless of presenting complaint. Knowing the reason Mr. D. did not go to see the doctor or knowing his last blood glucose reading does not alter your priority actions at this point. **Focus:** Prioritization

2. **Ans: 5**   Mr. D. should be taken to a treatment room where evaluation and treatment can begin immediately. Paging the ED physician to triage is not necessary unless the client codes in the triage area. Calling the parents is not necessary because Mr. D. is old enough to sign consent for himself. (If Mr. D. were underage, the treatment would not be delayed if the parents were unavailable in an emergency situation.) Calling the primary care physician is usually done by the ED physician after the preliminary workup is completed. (Policies for calling private physicians vary among institutions.) **Focus:** Prioritization

3. **Ans: 3**   Mr. D. is severely dehydrated and is at risk for hypovolemic shock. Although he is demonstrating Kussmaul respirations, the breathing pattern is the body's attempt to compensate for the acidosis. Anxiety and noncompliance are also relevant, but can be

addressed after Mr. D.'s condition is stabilized. **Focus:** Prioritization

4. **Ans: 1, 2, 3, 5**   Vital signs, bagging up belongings, and measuring/recording output are within the scope of duties for the nursing assistant. Releasing information should not be done by the nursing assistant due to confidentiality issues. The RN should decide how to convey information to friends and family who are waiting. Checking blood glucose is usually accomplished with a fingerstick, which is not usually within the scope of practice for the nursing assistant. **Focus:** Delegation

5. **Ans: 1, 2, 5, 6**   Mr. D. needs IV fluids to correct fluid deficit. Urine output must be monitored hourly, and a Foley with urinometer is the most accurate method. Mr. D. should be kept in a semi- to high-Fowler's position to prevent aspiration if he vomits. Oxygen is provided because he is at risk for hypovolemic shock. Subcutaneous insulin does not absorb fast enough and is inappropriate for emergency situations. (IV insulin would be appropriate.) He is likely to be NPO (nothing by mouth) until the vomiting stops. **Focus:** Prioritization

6. **Ans: 1**   Normal saline (0.9% sodium chloride) is the first fluid used to correct dehydration in most adults with DKA. Half-strength saline (0.45% sodium chloride) can be used for children or adults at risk for volume overload. Potassium supplements are added within 1–2 hours after starting insulin. Solutions of dextrose 5% are added to the therapy once the blood sugar approaches 250 mg/dL. **Focus:** Prioritization

7. **Ans: 2**   Within the first 4 hours of starting treatment in clients with DKA, you expect to see a serum potassium level that is within normal limits or elevated. Within 4–24 hours you would expect hypokalemia as the potassium shifts back into the cells. **Focus:** Prioritization

8. **Ans: 7, 2, 6, 4, 5, 3, 1**   An IV bolus of regular insulin is given first. Next, prime the tubing with normal saline prior to adding the insulin because the insulin will adhere to the tubing. After the tubing is flushed, draw up 100 units of regular insulin and have another nurse double check the amount and type. Add the insulin to 100 mL of normal saline to create a 1:1 solution. Label the bag clearly with the amount and type of insulin. (Hospital policies may vary to include your name, time, and date.) Insulin drips should always be delivered through a pump. The standard dose begins at 0.1 unit/kg/hr. **Focus:** Prioritization

9. **Ans: 2**   Ask the secretary to correct the omission by calling the admissions office right away. In this case, client care is more urgent than filing a complaint or determining why the secretary made the omission. If you have a good relationship with the ICU nurses, they will probably take report; however, you retain responsibility for care until the admission procedure and transfer are completed. **Focus:** Supervision

10. **Ans: 1, 4, 5, 6**   The nursing assistant can direct family and visitors to appropriate waiting areas, obtain equipment, and do vitals signs. An RN or MD should accompany Mr. D. to the ICU; the nursing assistant can help, but should not independently transport clients to the ICU. The unit secretary usually prepares the papers, but the RN is responsible for ensuring that everything is in order. Depending on the organization's job description, additional training may be done so that nursing assistants or technicians may place Mr. D. on the

monitor. Placing Mr. D. on the cardiac monitor may be done by the experienced nursing assistant, but the RN is responsible for assessing the cardiac rhythm. **Focus:** Delegation

Case Study 6: Home Health, pages 115–119

1. **Ans: Ms. A., Mr. F., Ms. I., Ms. R.**   Ms. A's dyspnea and use of increased oxygen require rapid assessment. Ms. F. is due for the epoetin injection. Mr. I.'s CBC must be drawn when the bone marrow is most suppressed to accurately assess the impact of chemotherapy on bone marrow function. Ms. R. should be seen as soon as possible after discharge in order to determine the plan of care. Mr. D. and Mr. S. do not have urgent needs and can be re-scheduled for the following day. **Focus:** Prioritization

2. **Ans: 1**   Ms. A.'s increased shortness of breath indicates a need for rapid assessment. In addition, high oxygen flow rates can suppress respiratory drive in patients with COPD, so Ms. A. should be seen as soon as possible. The other patients can be scheduled according to criteria such as location or patient preference about visit time. **Focus:** Prioritization

3. **Ans: 4**   In the home health setting, the patient is in control of health management, so enlisting the patient's cooperation for the visit is essential. In this response, the nurse indicates that the patient has a choice about whether the visit is scheduled for today, but educates the patient about why it is important that the visit occur as soon as possible. Because the initial visit requires a multi-dimensional assessment, it is usually quite lengthy. The patient's comments do not indicate a lack of need or desire for home health services. **Focus:** Prioritization

4. **Ans: 2**   The patient has symptoms and risk factors that could indicate that her oxygen saturation is either excessively high or too low, so checking oxygen saturation is the first action that should be taken. The other actions may also be appropriate, but assessment of oxygen saturation will determine which action should occur next. **Focus:** Prioritization

5. **Ans: 1**   The goal for oxygen saturation for a patient with COPD is usually about 90% to 92%, because high oxygen levels suppress respiratory drive and lead to increases in $Paco_2$. You should then notify the physician, who may want to admit the patient to the hospital or obtain arterial blood gas (ABG) values. It will be important to discuss appropriate home oxygen use with the patient and her husband, but not until the immediate situation is resolved. **Focus:** Prioritization

6. **Ans: Ms. F.**   Although ideally it would be best to administer the epoetin today, there will be little impact on the patient's chronic anemia if she receives the medication tomorrow. The other doses that are due this week can be rescheduled. **Focus:** Prioritization

7. **Ans: 2**   The chest pressure indicates that Ms. R. is experiencing myocardial ischemia and requires immediate assessment and intervention (such as sublingual nitroglycerin). The shortness of breath requires further investigation and may be related to the chest pressure and myocardial ischemia. The other responses also indicate the need for further assessment and interventions, such as teaching, but do not require immediate action. **Focus:** Prioritization

8. **Ans: 3**   If the patient is having any evidence of continued myocardial ischemia, nitroglycerin sublingual

tablets or spray should be used every 5 minutes for three doses. If the pain persists after three nitroglycerin tablets are given, the patient should be transported to the emergency department, because it is likely that an acute myocardial infarction is occurring. Completing the admission assessment, having her rest, and notifying the physician about her chest pain are also appropriate actions, but administration of another nitroglycerin tablet and resolution of the chest pressures are the priorities. **Focus:** Prioritization

9. **Ans: 4, 5, 6** Home health aide education and scope of practice include assisting with personal hygiene and obtaining routine data such as vital signs and daily weights. It is the RN's responsibility to evaluate these data and plan individualized care using the data. The other assessments and interventions require RN-level education and scope of practice. **Focus:** Delegation

10. **Ans: 2** The focus in home health nursing is empowering the patient and family members through teaching self-care. Ms. R.'s condition is not so unstable that she needs to be re-assessed today, since her chest pain did resolve after taking two nitroglycerin tablets, she has taken her medications, and her daughter will be available and has been educated about how to manage if Ms. R.'s condition deteriorates. The patient's symptoms of chest pressure, crackles, and edema do indicate a need for re-assessment the next day. Although the home health aide (HHA) will visit, HHA education and role do not include evaluating the patient's response to the ordered therapies and planning changes in care based on the evaluation. **Focus:** Prioritization

11. **Ans: Mr. I.** Because Mr. I. is in the nadir period following his chemotherapy, he is at high risk for infection. Avoidance of any cross-contamination from Mr. D.'s leg infection is essential. **Focus:** Prioritization

12. **Ans: 4** The initial assessment and development of the plan for care, including interventions such as oxygen therapy, are the responsibility of RN staff members. The RN with the most experience in caring for patients with emphysema is the on-call part-time RN. Some patient care activities are assigned to staff members from other disciplines such as LPNs and respiratory therapists after the plan of care is developed by the RN. **Focus:** Assignment

13. **Ans: 3** Immunosuppression decreases the patient's ability to mount a fever in response to infection, so that even a minor increase in temperature (especially in combination with symptoms such as lethargy and confusion) can be an indicator of a serious infection, including sepsis. The decreased right-sided breath sounds are consistent with the patient's diagnosis of lung cancer. The poor appetite and dry oral mucous membranes also require assessment and intervention, but infection is one of the most serious complications of chemotherapy. **Focus:** Prioritization

14. **Ans: 4** Mr. I.'s immunosuppression, fever, and possible sepsis diagnosis indicate that he should be assessed immediately once he arrives in the ED, so that he will avoid exposure to other ED patients. In addition, the appropriate treatment for sepsis is rapid initiation of IV antibiotics (after appropriate cultures are obtained). The other assessment information will also be helpful, but will not ensure that Mr. I is seen rapidly by the ED physician. A CBC will be obtained as part of the baseline laboratory assessment, based on Mr. I.'s diagnosis and chemotherapy treatment. **Focus:** Prioritization

15. **Ans: 2** All of the listed data indicate a need for assessment and/or intervention, especially the elevated temperature, but the elevated glucose would typically be treated immediately with administration of a rapid-acting insulin to prevent the development of serious complications such as diabetic ketoacidosis or hyperosmolar nonketotic coma. **Focus:** Prioritization

16. **Ans: 2, 3, 5, 6, 8, 9** The assessment on Mr. D. suggests that he has an acute lower respiratory tract infection such as pneumonia. The appropriate collaborative interventions for this include sputum culture and antibiotic therapy. Blood cultures are frequently ordered for patients with pneumonia, because sepsis is a possible complication. There are no data to suggest the need for urine or wound cultures. Daily oximetry is appropriate. Incentive spirometry and an increased fluid intake will both help loosen secretions. Since the patient is alert and is not hypoxemic or acutely dyspneic, he does not appear to require hospitalization at this time. You will want to reassess him the next day. **Focus:** Prioritization

Case Study 7: Spinal Cord Injury, pages 121–123

1. **Ans: 2** The priority at this time, with a C4-5 level spinal cord injury (SCI), is airway and respiratory status. The cervical spine nerves (C3-5) innervate the phrenic nerve, which controls the diaphragm. Careful and frequent assessments are necessary and endotracheal intubation may be necessary to prevent respiratory arrest. The other three concerns are appropriate, but are not urgent, as are airway and respiratory status. **Focus:** Prioritization

2. **Ans: 2, 4** The experienced nursing assistant can make sure that the oxygen flow setting is correct and that the cannula is in place once instructed by the RN. The experienced nursing assistant would also know how to measure oxygen saturation by pulse oximetry. The nurse retains responsibility for assuring that the client's oxygen flow rate is correct and for interpretation of oxygen saturation measurements. Assessments, including auscultation, and client teaching require additional education, training, and skill and are appropriate to the scope of practice for the professional RN. **Focus:** Delegation/supervision

3. **Ans: 3** The nurse should notify the physician immediately. The client's symptoms indicate the strong possibility of impending respiratory arrest. This client probably needs endotracheal intubation and mechanical ventilation. **Focus:** Prioritization

4. **Ans: 1** The traction weights must be hanging freely at all times to maintain the cervical traction and prevent further injury. All of the other actions are appropriate for the care of a client with cervical tongs. **Focus:** Prioritization

5. **Ans: 1, 4** A nursing student can administer medications and simple treatments such as cervical tong pin care. The nursing student should be mentored by the nurse when monitoring traction during client repositioning and performing neurologic assessments. **Focus:** Delegation/supervision

6. **Ans: 1** The experienced nursing assistant has been taught how to reposition clients, while maintaining proper body alignment. The nurse remains responsible for ensuring that this action is performed correctly. Inspecting clients' skin and administering medications require additional education and skill, appropriate to licensed nurses. Performing ROM exercise also requires

additional education and skill and is appropriate to the scope of practice of licensed nurses and physical therapists. However, some nursing assistants are given extra training and are able to perform ROM exercises for clients. Check the skill level and job description of your nursing assistant team members to determine their ability to perform ROM. **Focus:** Delegation/supervision

7. **Ans: 3** Mr. M. has a level C4-5 spinal injury. The best way to assess motor functions in a client with this level injury is to apply downward pressure while the client shrugs his shoulders upward. Testing plantar flexion assesses S1 level injuries. Application of resistance when client lifts his or her legs assesses L2-4 level injuries. Having a client grasp and form a fist assesses C8 level injuries. **Focus:** Prioritization

8. **Ans: 3** The client should be encouraged to perform as much self-care as he is able, and the nursing assistant should help with care the client is unable to complete. The client's wife should also be taught to encourage the client to do as much as possible for himself. **Focus:** Prioritization, delegation

9. **Ans: 1, 2, 3, 4, 5, 6** Clients should be taught to drink 2000–2500 mL of fluid each day to prevent urinary tract infections and calculus formations. They may be taught to decrease the amount of fluid intake after 6–7 PM to decrease the need to void or to self-catheterize in the middle of the night. The other points are appropriate to a bladder training program. **Focus:** Prioritization

10. **Ans: 2** The first, third, and fourth statements are reasonable client goals for rehabilitation. The second statement is probably an unrealistic expectation, and the client needs additional teaching about setting realistic goals for rehabilitation. **Focus:** Prioritization

Case Study 8: Multiple Patients with Adrenal Gland Disorders, pages 125–128

1. **Ans: 3** These signs and symptoms indicate adrenal crisis (Addisonian crisis), acute adrenocortical insufficiency, which is a life-threatening event in which the need for cortisol and aldosterone is greater than the available supply. The other actions are important and will likely be implemented rapidly because a common cause of acute adrenal gland hypofunction is hemorrhage, but the physician must be notified immediately. **Focus:** Prioritization

2. **Ans: 1** The patient is hypotensive and most likely hypovolemic. Because the patient already has an IV line, begin the IV fluids first to respond to the primary problem. The second IV line and type and cross need to be accomplished rapidly, and the blood sample may be drawn at the same time the second IV line is inserted. The patient needs cortisol replacement, but with nausea and vomiting present, the oral route is not the best route. **Focus:** Prioritization

3. **Ans: 2, 3, 4** The patient is experiencing nausea and vomiting so oral fluids are not appropriate at this time. The nursing assistant can take frequent vital signs, record intake and output, and weigh the patient. The nurse should instruct the nursing assistant about what variations in vital signs must be reported. **Focus:** Delegation/supervision

4. **Ans: 1** The manifestations the patient has developed are classic signs of hypoglycemia, a complication of adrenal gland hypofunction. The nurse should check the patient's glucose. If it is low, the patient should

receive some form of glucose, most likely dextrose 50% IV. **Focus:** Prioritization

5. **Ans: 4** The patient with hypercortisolism is immunosuppressed because excess cortisol reduces the number of circulating lymphocytes and inhibits production of cytokines and inflammatory chemicals such as histamine. These patients are at greater risk for infection. **Focus:** Prioritization

6. **Ans: 1** Women with hypercortisolism may report a history of cessation of menses. Increased androgen production can interrupt the normal hormone feedback mechanism for the ovary, decreasing the production of estrogens and progesterone and resulting in oligomenorrhea (scant or infrequent menses). All of the other responses are typical of adrenal gland hypofunction (e.g., Addison's disease). Typically patients with Cushing's disease have weight gain and do not experience gastrointestinal symptoms. **Focus:** Prioritization

7. **Ans: 1, 3, 4** The patient with Cushing's disease typically has a weight gain as a result of an increase in total body fat due to slow turnover of plasma fatty acids. Weight loss is to be expected in the patient with hypocortisolism (e.g., Addison's disease). The other findings are typical of a patient with Cushing's disease. **Focus:** Supervision, prioritization

8. **Ans: 3, 4** The LPN/LVN's educational preparation includes fingerstick glucose monitoring and administration of subcutaneous medications. Assessing cardiac rhythms and reviewing laboratory results require additional education and skill appropriate to the RN's scope of practice. **Focus:** Delegation/supervision

9. **Ans: 1, 3** The nursing assistant can provide articles for self-care and reinforce what the RN has already taught the patient. The nursing assistant can also remind the patient about changing positions. Instructing and assessing are within the scope of practice for the professional nurse. **Focus:** Delegation/supervision

10. **Ans: 1, 3, 4, 5, 6** Cortisol replacement therapy should be taken with meals or snacks because the patient can develop gastrointestinal irritation when the drugs (cortisone, hydrocortisone, prednisone, fludrocortisone) are taken on an empty stomach. All of the other teaching points are appropriate. **Focus:** Prioritization

11. **Ans: 3** Increased aldosterone levels affect the renal tubules and cause sodium retention with potassium and hydrogen ion excretion. Sodium retention results in increased retention of water and increased blood volume and pressure. Excretion of potassium places the patient at risk for the side effects of hypokalemia including cardiac dysrhythmias. Problems with hypokalemia and elevated blood pressure are most common with this condition. **Focus:** Prioritization

12. **Ans: 1** When assessing a patient with possible pheochromocytoma, do not palpate the abdomen because this action could cause a sudden release of catecholamines and severe hypertension. None of the other assessments should have an adverse effect on this patient. **Focus:** Prioritization

13. **Ans: 3** During the 3–4 day VMA testing period, medications usually withheld include aspirin and antihypertensive agents. Beta blockers are avoided because these drugs may cause a rebound rise in blood pressure. All of the other instructions are appropriate for this diagnostic test. **Focus:** Delegation/supervision

14. **Ans: 2** The nursing assistant should remind the patient about elements of the care regimen that

the nurse has already taught the patient. Assessing, instructing, and identifying stressful situations that may trigger a hypertensive crisis require additional education and skill appropriate to the scope of practice of the professional RN. **Focus:** Delegation/supervision

15. **Ans: 1, 4** The new graduate nurse who has just completed orientation should be assigned patients whose conditions are relatively stable and not complex. The new graduate should be familiar with the adrenal surgery after completing her orientation and should be able to provide the teaching the patient needs. The patient with a low potassium level will need some form of potassium supplementation, which the new nurse should be able to administer. The patient with Addisonian crisis should be assigned to an experienced nurse. The fearful, anxious patient would also benefit from being assigned to an experienced nurse. **Focus:** Assignment

Case Study 9: Multiple Clients with Gastrointestinal Problems, pages 129—133

1. **Ans: 1, 3, 4** Ms. H., Ms. D., and Mr. A. are the most stable and least complex cases according to the shift report. Mr. R.'s anxiety and belligerence will make pain management especially difficult. Because of his pancreatitis, laboratory results should be closely monitored. Ms. T. is at risk for electrolyte imbalances, especially hypokalemia. She needs repetitive perineal hygiene and skin assessment. TPN and central line management require additional skill. Mr. K. is stable, but the family dynamics should be handled by an experienced nurse. **Focus:** Assignment

2. **Ans: 2** When the shift report is incomplete, you can ask for any type of additional information. However, vital signs and orders for medications can be obtained from the records if the off-going shift neglects to give that information. A current pain assessment can and should be obtained directly from the client. The physician's plan for procedures and diagnostic testing is frequently communicated verbally to the nursing staff, but the notes may be pending, especially in the case of an emergency admission or if the physician is trying to complete morning rounds. **Focus:** Prioritization

3. **Ans: 1, 3, 2, 4** Mr. R. is having severe pain, and elevations in WBC and glucose are two indicators associated with increased mortality rates for clients with pancreatitis. Ms. T. should be monitored for fluid and electrolyte imbalances. Ms. D. needs a pain assessment, and IV site should be evaluated. Mr. A. is stable. **Focus:** Prioritization

4. **Ans: 1** In providing routine care, clients who need extra time should be left until last, so that care for others is not delayed. Mr. K. will require more time and assistance because of age and weakness. Dealing with Mr. K.'s family is also more time consuming. **Focus:** Prioritization

5. **Ans: 1, 2, 3, 4** Vital signs, hygienic care, and transporting are within the scope of the nursing assistant's duties. The nursing assistant could also take the dressing materials to Mr. A.'s room; however, you will have to give her a list of items. Mr. A. has asked for additional instructions about dressing changes, and you could easily combine the teaching with delivering the materials. In delegating duties, you must consider the complexity of each task and the overall efficient use of personnel. **Focus:** Delegation

6. **Ans: 3, 4** Nursing assistants can report on changes in vital signs; giving parameters is better than asking for general reports on any changes. The nursing assistant can report that the client is having pain, but is not expected to assess that pain. Skin assessment and evaluation of drainage are responsibilities of the RN. Nursing assistants are often instructed to report any changes in skin condition that they may note throughout the shift subsequent to the RN's initial skin assessment. **Focus:** Delegation

7. **Ans: 1** Meperidine (Demerol) has traditionally been the drug of choice. Morphine may cause spasm in the sphincter of Oddi. Other options that have been used successfully to manage acute pain in clients with pancreatitis include transdermal fentanyl and epidural morphine with bupivacaine. Lortab and Darvocet are given for mild to moderate pain. **Focus:** Prioritization/ knowledge

8. **Ans: 3** Giving written information about GB disease and options will help her to prepare any questions she might have for the doctor. If diagnostic results are pending, calling the physician is premature. Describing the surgical procedure is inappropriate because there is more than one type of procedure, and the decision is yet undetermined. Demonstrating coughing and deep breathing will not hurt her, but does nothing to relieve her concerns about the surgical process. **Focus:** Prioritization

9. **Ans: 4** Stopping the diarrhea is a priority for Ms. T. Chronic, frequent diarrhea is demoralizing, and fluid and electrolyte losses cause weakness. If the bowel is allowed to rest, the cramping will stop. The other options are also accurate information, but the potential resolution of the most disturbing symptoms will encourage her to continue. **Focus:** Prioritization

10. **Ans: 3** Sulfasalazine is potentially nephrotoxic. The other adverse effects are also possible, but less serious. **Focus:** Prioritization

11. **Ans: 4** Explaining the physiologic reason to the nursing assistant helps her to understand that rest is part of the therapy. Following doctor's orders is important, but it is an inadequate explanation. Depression does not justify bedrest. Using large words to explain common concepts should be avoided regardless of the audience. **Focus:** Supervision

12. **Ans: 2** Bowel sounds should resume in 24 hours; this signals GI system readiness. The client's subjective reports of hunger (or lack of hunger) should not dictate initiation of feedings. The pharmacy may label the formula according to the prescriber's order, but will not determine the feeding schedule. **Focus:** Prioritization

13. **Ans: 1, 3, 4** Elderly clients are especially at risk for hyperglycemia, aspiration, and diarrhea. Hypertension is not a direct complication of enteral feedings. **Focus:** Prioritization

14. **Ans: 1, 3, 2, 4, 1** Instruct the nursing assistant to hold direct pressure on Ms. D.'s IV site until the bleeding stops. Use therapeutic communication skills with Mr. R.; he is at risk for injury and self-harm. He must be assessed for mental status changes related to decision-making. Assess Ms. H.'s vomiting and give an antiemetic if appropriate. Assess what Mr. K.'s family needs from the doctor and page the doctor if appropriate. Return to Ms. D.'s room and restart her IV. **Focus:** Prioritization/delegation

15. **Ans: 4** Helping her to prioritize will build skill and confidence. She feels upset, but she has not made any errors that have compromised client care. Sending her off the unit further delays care, leaves her without support, and hinders opportunities to problem solve. Asking the nursing assistant to help her or helping her with select tasks is the second best choice because it demonstrates team support. Taking over one of her clients is not necessary unless care and safety are compromised. **Focus:** Supervision

16. **Ans: 1** If Mr. A. is homeless, he will need instructions for adapting the dressing change procedure or referral to a clinic. The social worker should be contacted for issues of no money for medication or transportation problems. Simplify written material and verbally reinforce and/or instruct Mr. A. to have a friend read the information to him. **Focus:** Prioritization

17. **Ans: 3** Washing the hands is the first basic step for dressing change. Helping him identify other ways to maintain asepsis would be more useful than stressing strict sterile technique. **Focus:** Prioritization

18. **Ans: 1, 2, 3, 4** The low calcium and the falling HCT and Po_2, in combination with the elevated WBC and his age are indicators of a high mortality rate. High level of pain is not a prognostic factor, but severe unrelieved pain should always be reported. **Focus:** Prioritization

19. **Ans: 3, 5, 4, 1, 6, 2, 7** Stay with the client and have a colleague gather equipment. (Note: If O_2 tubing/mask is available in the room, apply it immediately.) Restart the IV to give emergency fluids or drugs. Check blood sugar to rule out a hypoglycemic reaction. Place monitoring equipment and repeat vital signs. **Focus:** Prioritization

20. **Ans: 3** Mr. R. has sufficient criteria to warrant intensive care. The physician is responsible for the decision to transfer Mr. R. However, the nurse must recognize and advocate for clients who are decompensating. Ordering laboratory and other diagnostic testing may occur, such as reestablishing IV and NG tubes, and keeping the doctor informed, are appropriate until the definitive decision is made. Surgery is unlikely until aggressive medical management is exhausted. **Focus:** Prioritization

21. **Ans: 1, 3, 5, 6, 7** Transferring Mr. R. to ICU is a priority because he is unstable. Documentation must be completed, and totaling IV fluids is part of the complete documentation. Briefly assessing clients is a safety measure; client decompensation during shift change is not uncommon. Thanking ancillary staff is a team-building measure. Asking the nursing assistant to do vital signs on all the clients is unnecessary. If select clients are unstable, or if there is a reason that the vital signs may have changed since the last routine reading, then retaking vital signs is appropriate. Asking the ED to hold the client until the next shift will displease the ED staff, but the client deserves a thorough assessment and review of orders. The admission should be deferred to the oncoming shift, if the client is stable and has had immediate care needs met, unless there is adequate time to complete the task. **Focus:** Prioritization

Case Study 10: Multiple Patients with Pain, pages 135–138

1. **Ans: 6, 4, 2, 1, 5** Mr. A.'s respiratory status (i.e., rate, rhythm, pulse oximetry) should be quickly checked. Mr. O. should be checked for shock symptoms, mental status changes, and escalating pain. Mr. L. and Ms. R.
are both relatively safe, but need quick pain assessments and reassurance that their needs will be met. Ms. J. and her family should be approached last because they need time and patience, and caregivers should not appear rushed. Mr. H. is currently in the OR. **Focus:** Prioritization

2. **Ans: 1, 2, 3** Ms. R. and Mr. L. have conditions that require pain medication, but are less physiologically complex. Mr. H. will be newly post-operative later in the shift, but hernia repairs are routine and reasonably predictable; this is a good post-operative case for a new RN. Mr. O. will require careful assessment for slowly developing complications such as hemorrhage or peritonitis. Ms. J. and her family will need support through anticipated grief and loss and complex decision making for hospice and end of life issues. Mr. A.'s respiratory status must be carefully monitored and he has complex pain and care issues. **Focus:** Assignment

3. **Ans: 2** You should encourage staff members to first deal directly with each other to define and resolve problems. If staff cannot resolve the problem amongst themselves or if the issue is a chronic problem, then the charge nurse or unit manager should intervene. Helping the new nurse to look at the chart should not be necessary at this point. Asking the patient does not address the problem of the missing documentation. **Focus:** Supervision

4. **Ans: 1, 2, 3** Helping Ms. R. with hygienic care is appropriate. After shoulder arthroplasty, she will be unable to do it herself. The nursing assistant can reinforce instructions to Mr. L. that have been explained by the RN. Mr. H. should not need any specialized equipment, so the nursing assistant can tidy the room, prepare the bed, and so on. Mr. O.'s skin care and assessment should be done by the RN; the problem is extensive and pain medication may need to be titrated. Ms. J.'s family should be encouraged to take occasional breaks off the floor. Sending one of the family members to get things is a way for them to have an active role. **Focus:** Delegation

5. **Ans: 1, 3, 5** Because communication in unresponsive patients is limited, all staff members should be watchful for signs. The RN should instruct the nursing assistant on specific things to watch for. Reminding patients that staff are available to help relieve pain is appropriate. If the nursing assistant suspects pain, asking the patient a direct yes or no question is appropriate; then the nurse can be notified. Assessing the pain and evaluating outcomes are the responsibility of the RN. **Focus:** Delegation

6. **Ans: 3** Elevating the injured extremity will minimize the swelling. If the leg swells, there is additional pressure on nerves. Moving the toes helps, but use of opioids will make Mr. O. very sleepy. Diversional therapy is less useful in the acute phase of injury and treatment. Placing him in high-Fowler's position will necessitate raising the leg to a higher and more uncomfortable position. **Focus:** Prioritization

7. **Ans: 1** Pain on passive motion is a sign of possible compartment syndrome. Sudden increase in pain is more associated with arterial obstruction. Pain with dorsiflexion is one of the signs of deep vein thrombosis. Pain free without medication could be related to maintaining elevation, ice, and rest. **Focus:** Prioritization

8. **Ans: 3** Mr. L. is having an exacerbation of pain that is probably related to the movement of the kidney stone.

This type of pain is severe, but usually transient. If the bolus dose is inadequate, the physician could be notified for a dosage increase. Deep breathing may help somewhat, but he will have trouble focusing. Reminding him to use the PCA is not necessary at this point. **Focus:** Prioritization

9. **Ans: 2**   Mr. H. is anticipating that the pain is going to be worsened by the activity. Giving medication 45 minutes before the activity assures him that the pain will be minimized. The second best option is to reassure him that medication is available if he needs it. Around-the-clock medication and notifying the physician are not necessary at this point. **Focus:** Prioritization/knowledge

10. **Ans: 2, 4, 1, 4 3, 2**   It is unlikely that Ms. J.'s pump will deliver excess medication; however, it is appropriate to quickly turn it off until the function can be completely checked. Delegate the nursing assistant to help Mr. A. back into bed. Mr. L. is probably having ongoing pain issues, but loud calls for assistance must be investigated. Mr. A. must be assessed for mental status changes related to hypoxia or encephalopathy. The other nurse could ask someone else to witness if necessary. Go back and troubleshoot Ms. J.'s PCA pump. **Focus:** Prioritization

11. **Ans: 4**   Mr. A. has complex needs. Although the staff gets tired of hearing continuous complaints, everyone should work together to try and solve the problem. Reminding staff that patients have a right to care is rhetorical and not very useful. Offering to take Mr. A. everyday does not help the team to overcome bias or improve patient care. When giving feedback, statements that begin with "You should" should be avoided. **Focus:** Supervision

12. **Ans: 1. PT, 2. RN, 3. RN, 4. PT, 5. RN, 6. NA**   TENS and ultrasound require specialized equipment and training and should be handled by a physical therapist. An RN should give medications and answer questions. Personal comfort items are permissible, but the RN should remind the family that belongings can get misplaced. The nursing assistant is qualified to help with routine position changes. **Focus:** Assignment

13. **Ans: 3**   He may be having urinary retention due to bladder atony related to the surgical procedure. A distended bladder can mimic hernia pain and cause significant discomfort, and Mr. H. may not have the urge to void. Calling the physician and making the patient NPO are premature at this point. Reassurance may be somewhat comforting, but does not solve the immediate symptom. **Focus:** Prioritization

14. **Ans: 3**   Scant output suggests that the stone is lodged and obstructing the outflow of urine. This can result in damage to the kidney. Hematuria with or without pain can occur because the stone has irritated the tissue. Dull pain that radiates into the genitalia and urgency are common with stones. **Focus:** Prioritization

15. **Ans: 2**   If you decide to question the nurse or check on the patients, specific examples are more useful than vague generalizations. Specific examples will also help you determine whether there are extenuating circumstances that the nursing assistant may be misinterpreting. Comments about patient care issues should not be ignored; all team members should be encouraged to watch out for the health and safety of the patients. **Focus:** Supervision

16. **Ans: 1**   Ms. J. has been receiving opiates for an extended period of time. Constipation is the only opi-

oid side effect that is not subject to tolerance. Respiratory depression, nausea, vomiting, and sedation may have occurred when Ms. J. was first getting opioids, but are now less of a concern. **Focus:** Prioritization

17. **Ans: 3**   Lorazepam is an anxiolytic. Naproxen sodium is an NSAID. Doxepin hydrochloride is used for depression or neuropathic pain. Dicyclomine hydrochloride is for smooth muscle spasms. **Focus:** Prioritization/knowledge

18. **Ans: 4**   Communication skills are important in handling the family and the doctor. If you have exhausted this route, the next step is to follow the chain of command. Calling another physician is not appropriate. If the son calls the doctor, it may make the situation worse. You must function under the current orders and use additional non-pharmaceutical measures until the issue is resolved. **Focus:** Prioritization

19. **Ans: 3**   Help the nurse prioritize what has to be done, and help her recognize what can and cannot be delegated. Offering help is appropriate if patient safety is compromised, and it does contribute to team building; however, it does not help her to learn to organize her work. Letting her struggle is one method of learning, but she may not realize that it is okay to let the oncoming shift assume the care of the patient. **Focus:** Supervision

Case Study 11: Multiple Clients with Cancer, pages 139–142

1. **Ans: 1, 2, 5, 6**   When the client responds to a question, you gather information about ease of respirations and cerebral perfusion. Noting presence of complex equipment will help in making assignments, particularly if the staff is inexperienced. Taking vital signs, checking I&O, and palpating for pain are not necessary during this brief assessment, unless there is reason to suspect that the client is decompensating. (Note: Some nurses will briefly palpate radial pulse to detect irregularities and assess peripheral perfusion.) **Focus:** Prioritization

2. **Ans: 2, 3, 4**   Mr. N., Mr. B., and Ms. C. are relatively stable clients who would be capable of speaking with a nursing student for a prolonged time. Mr. L. is a recent transfer from SICU. His tracheostomy tube with secretions and the NG tube will make communication very tedious and overwhelming for him and the student. Mr. U. needs continuous assessment on the first postoperative day, and he is likely to be very uncomfortable, exhausted, and possibly dyspneic. Ms. G. needs emotional support and pre-operative teaching that are beyond the abilities of a first-semester student. **Focus:** Assignment

3. **Ans: 2**   Staff and visitors with potentially communicable diseases should not enter Mr. N.'s protective environment. Pregnancy, inexperience, and fear do not automatically exclude staff members from this assignment. If the team leader has time and options for personnel, then opportunities for duty sharing for pregnant staff members and teaching the inexperienced and fearful can be explored. **Focus:** Assignment

4. **Ans: 4**   Increased secretions, difficulty swallowing, and loss of the protective epiglottis put Mr. L. at risk for aspiration. The other diagnoses also apply to this client, but are of lower priority. **Focus:** Prioritization

5. **Ans: 1**   Frank bleeding is not expected and may signal hemorrhage from the surgical site or eroding of the

adjacent vessels. The other options are expected in the post-operative period for a tracheostomy. **Focus:** Prioritization

6. **Ans: 2, 3, 5, 6, 7** Insertion of suppositories (probes or tampons) into the rectal (or vaginal) cavity is not recommended. Mouthwash should not include alcohol because it has a drying action that leaves mucous membranes more vulnerable. All other options are appropriate. **Focus:** Prioritization/knowledge

7. **Ans: 2, 3, 1, 4, 6, 5** A Foley catheter with a drainage bag will be inserted. The BCG fluid is instilled through the catheter, and then the catheter is clamped for 2 hours. During those hours, Mr. B. should be reminded to change position side to side or prone to supine every 15–30 minutes. At the end of the 2 hours, the catheter is unclamped, and the fluid is drained. Two glasses of fluid are given to further flush the bladder. **Focus:** Prioritization

8. **Ans: 3** The toilet should be disinfected for 6 hours after discarding the fluid. The nursing assistant should receive these specific instructions to safely manage this biohazard. Wearing a lead apron and sterile gloves are not necessary. **Focus:** Delegation

9. **Ans: 3** The goal is resumption of normal voiding within 3 days. Immediately after catheter removal and for 2 days thereafter, Mr. B. may experience dysuria, urgency, and frequency. **Focus:** Prioritization

10. **Ans: 4, 2, 3, 5, 1** Mr. L. is at risk for aspiration and an immediate airway obstruction if he is not suctioned. If a chest drainage system does tip over, it is unlikely that anything untoward will occur; however, if the chest tube has been displaced, Mr. U. is at risk for an open pneumothorax. The physician must be notified about Mr. N. for a change in therapy and orders for cultures to determine the source of infection. Ms. C. must be assessed for signs of deep vein thrombosis. Mr. B. needs reassurance that the dysuria is transient and to be expected after intravesical therapy. **Focus:** Delegation/prioritization

11. **Ans: 3** Acknowledge the student for taking responsibility for the error. Helping the student to feel comfortable in reporting errors rather than hiding mistakes is essential for client safety. Notifying the instructor is appropriate so that the student can be counseled and procedures reviewed. All involved parties may elect to write separate incident reports. **Focus:** Supervision

12. **Ans: 1. NA, 2. RN, 3. RN, 4. ET, 5. ET** The nursing assistant is able to assist Ms. C. with toileting needs. The RN should explain the need for a rectal dressing and give medications. An enterostomal therapist, if available, is best qualified to answer questions about the ostomy and stoma placement. **Focus:** Assignment

13. **Ans: 4** Asking for extra help and delaying independent action is a type of regression that allows Ms. C. to cope with the changes in self-image and bodily functions. The nurse should evaluate the situation daily to help Ms. C. find alternative coping strategies. The other diagnoses may be relevant as her situation changes. **Focus:** Prioritization

14. **Ans: 4** Have her hold the clamp or do some other small task to engage her in participation. This creates the expectation that she can participate and will eventually handle the equipment. Verbally re-explaining the procedure and written material does reinforce the initial teaching, but being told will not help her master the psychomotor aspects. Having a family member or a staff member take over the procedure does not support the goal of eventual independence. **Focus:** Prioritization

15. **Ans: 1** Ms. G. is demonstrating fear and anxiety related to the unknown. The other diagnoses are pertinent, but getting the anxiety under control precedes giving her information, decision making, or dealing with body image. **Focus:** Prioritization

16. **Ans: 1** All of the conditions warrant calling the physician. However, tracheal deviation is a symptom of tension pneumothorax, and the nurse may have to intervene before the physician can arrive or phone in orders. Dysrhythmias are one sign of tumor lysis syndrome secondary to hyperkalemia. A pulsating tracheostomy tube may mean that it is resting on a major artery and has a potential for damage and hemorrhage. Ms. C. is at risk for hemorrhage or peritonitis. **Focus:** Prioritization

17. **Ans:** Any three of these seven additional assessment finds: severe dyspnea, extreme agitation, increased respiratory rate, increased pulse, progressive cyanosis, distended jugular veins, and lateral or median PMI shift. **Focus:** Prioritization

18. **Ans: 1** For Mr. U., the most likely cause of the tension pneumothorax is the iatrogenically induced covering of the chest wound. (For clients without open chest wounds, the priority action is a needle thoracotomy.) Initiating CPR is inappropriate at this point. Having the crash cart and intubation equipment nearby is a precaution, but should not delay other interventions. **Focus:** Prioritization

Case Study 12: Gastrointestinal Bleeding, pages 143–145

1. **Ans: 3** Vomiting bright red blood is a sign of active bleeding. The patient's physical assessment and vital signs are indicative of physiologic compensation for blood loss. Risk for aspiration is not an eminent concern because he is currently alert and there is no reason to suspect that his gag reflex is not intact. Anxiety and noncompliance can be addressed later. **Focus:** Prioritization

2. **Ans: 2, 3, 4, 5** Mr. S. is at risk for hypovolemic shock. Decreases in urine output or hemoglobin or hematocrit should be monitored. Hemoccult of emesis and stool should be performed to validate upper and lower GI bleeding. Semi- or high-Fowler's is used to decrease risk for aspiration during vomiting and/or NG tube insertion. A 22-gauge catheter is not the best choice for this patient. He may require a blood transfusion and/or large fluid volumes; 16- to 18-gauge catheters are better choices. Preparing the patient for surgery at this point is premature, because bleeding resolves spontaneously in most hospitalized patients. **Focus:** Prioritization

3. **Ans: 1** Repeating vital signs falls within the scope of the nursing assistant's abilities. Whereas checking the blood glucose is a task that the nursing assistant can perform, there is no indication that the patient needs this. Gathering certain types of equipment can be delegated. However, NG lavage is not a task of a nursing assistant; if you delegate this task, you will have to provide an itemized list. The nursing assistant should not be responsible for notification of the family, even with the patient's permission. **Focus:** Delegation

4. **Ans: 1. NA, 2. Paramedic or RN, 3. RN, 4. LPN/LVN, 5. RN, 6. Clergy, 7. RN** In an emergency situation, many team members under the supervision of the RN will perform tasks simultaneously, and there will

be variation and overlap among institutions for the roles and duties of personnel. The nursing assistant is capable of obtaining vital signs. Either an RN or a paramedic can insert peripheral IVs. NG and lavage should be done by the RN because the initial gastric return and response to lavage should be continuously assessed. Foley insertion can be done by the LPN/LVN. (Note: Some institutions will allow nursing assistants to insert Foleys with additional training.) Clergy (if available) can assist by comforting and supporting family members. If clergy is unavailable, the RN must assume this responsibility. Assessment should be performed by the RN. **Focus:** Assignment

5. **Ans: 3**   A tense, rigid abdomen could signal perforation, peritonitis, and/or a worsening hemorrhage. The other findings are relevant, but less immediately urgent. **Focus:** Prioritization

6. **Ans: 2, 1, 6, 7, 4, 3, 5**   Place the patient in high-Fowler's position to prevent aspiration. The length is measured for tip placement into the stomach. Check for the most patent nostril by inspecting or by occluding each nostril and checking for air flow. (Note: Checking for nostril patency could precede measuring the length of the tube.) Insert the tube into the most patent nostril and ask the patient to tip chin down, then gently advance the tube. When the tip reaches the posterior pharynx, have the patient sip water. Swallowing closes the epiglottis and helps to prevent tracheal intubation. Checking placement is essential prior to instilling saline. **Focus:** Prioritization

7. **Ans: 4**   Page the physician and document your actions. The physician may opt to order restraints if the situation is life-threatening and the patient is not coherent enough to make safe decisions. The physician may decide to talk to the patient and then have him sign an AMA form if the patient continues to refuse treatment. The nursing supervisor and the patient advocate can be notified if the situation escalates. **Focus:** Prioritization

8. **Ans: 2**   To expedite the STAT order, draw the specimen yourself. (In addition, you may delegate the unit clerk to call the laboratory and alert them to the error in labeling.) The other options will only delay the STAT order. After Mr. S. is stabilized, tracking down the cause of the error will help prevent recurrences. **Focus:** Prioritization/supervision

9. **Ans: 1**   In a medical emergency, the patient could receive O-negative (or O-positive) blood. Women should receive O negative only to prevent potential Rh incompatibilities in any future pregnancies. An antibody reaction could result if A or B blood types are administered without type and cross-match. **Focus:** Prioritization/knowledge

10. **Ans: 4, 5, 6, 1, 2, 3, 7, 8**   Inspect the bag. If the product appears unusable or if the bag is damaged, contact the blood bank for another unit. Checking labels and identification is essential. At the bedside, two licensed professionals should compare bag and ID band. (Note: Priming the tubing and filter could be done anytime prior to starting the transfusion. Many nurses will do this step while they are taking the vital signs with an automated BP cuff. In an emergency situation, equipment preparation can be done while waiting for the unit to come from the blood bank.) Taking vital signs immediately before starting the transfusion provides a baseline in case of transfusion reaction. The first 50

mL (or within 15 minutes) are the most likely to result in a reaction if it is going to occur. Frequent vital signs (according to hospital policy) and complete documentation are standard requirements. **Focus:** Prioritization

11. **Ans: 3**   Vasopressin is used to control acute and severe bleeding. Histamine H_2-receptor antagonists such as ranitidine or famotidine are used to decrease acid secretions. Other anti-ulcer drugs include antacids and proton-pump inhibitors. **Focus:** Prioritization/knowledge

Case Study 13: Head and Leg Trauma and Shock, pages 147–151

1. **Ans: 4**   Ms. A.'s slow and irregular respiratory rate is a risk factor for hypoxemia, which would decrease oxygen delivery to the brain as well as other vital organs and tissues. The other assessments should also be accomplished quickly because Ms. A. is at risk for hypothermia, blood loss associated with a possible left leg fracture, and aspiration. **Focus:** Prioritization

2. **Ans: 3**   The GCS offers a standardized and objective way to assess and document LOC. Although the other responses also accurately describe the client's LOC, they do not provide objective data that can be readily used to determine changes in the client's neurologic status. **Focus:** Prioritization

3. **Ans: Decerebrate**   Stiff extension of the arms and legs is seen in decerebrate posturing, which indicates damage to the midbrain and brainstem. **Focus:** Prioritization/knowledge

4. **Ans: 2, 3**   The usual response to hypotension is an increase in heart rate. Ms. A.'s bradycardia suggests that she is experiencing neurogenic shock in response to her head injury. It is also important to remember that with any traumatic injury, hypovolemic shock due to hemorrhage should be considered. In this case, Ms. A. should be assessed for blood loss associated with her leg injury and for internal bleeding caused by blunt trauma to her chest and abdomen. **Focus:** Prioritization

5. **Ans: 4**   Lumbar puncture is contraindicated in a client who may have increased intracranial pressure (ICP) because it increases the risk for herniation of the brainstem through the tentorial notch. Checking for a positive Babinski's sign and obtaining an ECG are not priorities for this client, but would not place the client at any increased risk. Increasing the IV rate is appropriate based on the client's blood pressure. **Focus:** Prioritization

6. **Ans: 3**   The initial care of clients with traumatic injuries in the ED requires the expertise of an RN with extensive ED experience. Neither the agency RN nor the intensive care RN will be familiar with the location of equipment and with the organization of care in your ED. Although the LPN/LVN has experience in the ED, LPN/LVN scope of practice does not include the complex assessments and interventions that will be needed in caring for this client. (The LPN/LVN could be assigned to assist the RN caring for Ms. A.) **Focus:** Assignment

7. **Ans: 1**   The most important goal for an unconscious client who is vomiting is to prevent aspiration. Turning Ms. A. to her side is the best method to ensure that Ms. A. does not aspirate. Suctioning would also be utilized, but does not clear the airway as well as having the client positioned on her side. Hyperoxygenation may also be required for this client, but will not protect the airway while she is vomiting. An NG tube is usually not inserted in clients with possible facial fractures. An oral-gastric

(OG) tube may be ordered, but would not protect from aspiration at the present time. **Focus:** Prioritization

8. **Ans: 4** Ms. A.'s arterial blood gases indicate uncompensated respiratory acidosis and hypoxemia. Because her respiratory drive is suppressed, she will need intubation and manual ventilation using a mechanical positive pressure ventilator. She may need surgery, in which case it would be appropriate to have blood available in the blood bank. Increasing her fluid rate may be needed based on her blood pressure, but is not indicated by her laboratory data. Insulin would not be administered for a small glucose elevation like this. **Focus:** Prioritization

9. **Ans: 2** The CT scan and x-rays are necessary to determine the collaborative interventions needed for this client, who may have chest, abdominal, and leg trauma that will require surgery in addition to her head injury. The other orders are also appropriate for the client, but do not need implementation as rapidly. **Focus:** Prioritization

10. **Ans: 1** The client's fixed and dilated pupils, widened pulse pressure, and bradycardia are caused by increasing pressure on the brain stem and indicate that she is at risk of herniation of the brain stem through the tentorial notch, which would result in brain death. Immediate surgical intervention is needed to prevent this complication. She is at risk for the other complications, but they are not as life-threatening. **Focus:** Prioritization

11. **Ans: 4** The cerebral perfusion pressure (CPP) should be maintained at 70 mm Hg or greater. CPP is calculated using the formula MAP – ICP = CPP. Ms. A.'s CPP is 54 mm Hg (71 – 17 = 54), so interventions should be implemented immediately to decrease her ICP. Interventions to increase Ms. A.'s MAP may also be used to improve her CPP. The other data indicate a need for ongoing monitoring, but do not require immediate intervention. **Focus:** Prioritization

12. **Ans: 1, 2, 7** The therapeutic effect of dexamethasone and mannitol for clients with increased ICP is to decrease cerebral edema. Positioning the head of the bed at 30 degrees also reduces cerebral edema by promoting venous drainage from the cerebral circulation. Although neurologic assessments such as checking the GCS and pupil reaction to light are necessary, the stimulation caused by these can increase ICP. In addition, suctioning and repositioning also cause transient increases in ICP. It is important to monitor ICP, MAP, and CPP during these procedures and modify care to avoid unnecessary increases in ICP or decreases in CPP. **Focus:** Prioritization

13. **Ans: 1, 6, 7, 8** Client data collection, collection of urine specimens, and administration of medications through an OG or NG tube are included in LPN/LVN education and scope of practice. An experienced LPN/LVN would be expected to report any changes in client status to the supervising RN. Usually repositioning a client would also be included in the LPN/LVN role; however, this client is at risk for increased ICP during positioning and should be monitored by the RN during and after repositioning. Assessments of breath sounds, neurologic status, and the endotracheal tube cuff in critically ill clients should be accomplished by an experienced RN. **Focus:** Delegation

14. **Ans: 1** Lower than normal $Paco_2$ levels cause cerebral vasoconstriction and result in further cerebral hypoxia. The RN should notify the physician and obtain an order to decrease the ventilator rate. The second priority is to decrease the Fio_2, since the Pao_2 and O_2 saturation indicate that Ms. A. does not need an Fio_2 of 60% to maintain adequate oxygenation. Prolonged use of an Fio_2 higher than 40% can lead to alveolar damage and acute respiratory distress syndrome (ARDS). The decrease in HCO_3 reflects a compensatory mechanism for the client's respiratory alkalosis and will resolve spontaneously when the $Paco_2$ level rises. **Focus:** Prioritization

15. **Ans: 3** Ms. A.'s high urine output suggests that she has developed diabetes insipidus (DI), a common complication of intracranial surgery. Because DI can rapidly lead to dehydration in a client who is unable to take in oral fluids, the priority action here is to obtain an order to increase the IV rate. Continuing to monitor the output and checking the specific gravity would also be needed, but would not correct the risk for dehydration. Since Ms. A.'s neurologic status is so poor, it is unlikely that changes in her neurologic status would be helpful in determining the effects of DI. **Focus:** Prioritization

16. **Ans: 2** Acute gastrointestinal bleeding caused by stress ulcers was a common complication of head injury until the development of H_2 blockers (such as famotidine) and proton-pump inhibitors (such as pantoprazole [Protonix]). Administration of famotidine may decrease the risk of pneumonitis if aspiration occurs, minimize the effects of gastroesophageal reflux, and decrease stomach irritation, but none of the other responses addresses the use of H_2 blockade in head injury. **Focus:** Prioritization

17. **Ans: 2** The head and neck should be maintained in good alignment, because neck flexion can cause venous obstruction and an increase in ICP. Administration of mannitol and further elevation of the head of the bed may be used to lower ICP if repositioning Ms. A.'s head and neck is ineffective. However, these should be used only if her MAP is high enough to maintain a CPP of 70 mm Hg. Checking Ms. A.'s pupils would not offer any additional information, and the stimulation may increase her ICP. **Focus:** Prioritization

18. **Ans: 1** Your assessment data point toward the complication of compartment syndrome, an emergency that can lead to permanent neuromuscular damage within 4–6 hours without rapid treatment. Elevation of the leg will further reduce blood flow to the leg. Continuing to monitor the leg and the client's neurologic status without correcting the compartment syndrome will allow the ischemia to persist. **Focus:** Prioritization

19. **Ans: 2** When a family member is available, the surgeon should obtain written permission from the family member after discussing the benefits and risks of the surgery. Emergency procedures can take place without written consent in an unconscious or incompetent client when no family or legal representative is available to give permission. The nursing supervisor does not have the authority to consent to surgery for an unconscious client. **Focus:** Prioritization

Case Study 14: Hypotension, Lethargy, Nausea, and Abdominal Pain, pages 153–157

1. **Ans: 2** The oxygen saturation indicates that the patient is severely hypoxic (despite an increased respiratory rate). Because this will affect all other body systems, it should be treated immediately. The other orders also should be rapidly implemented, but they

do not require action as urgently as the low oxygen saturation. **Focus:** Prioritization

2. **Ans: 2** A non-rebreather mask can provide an FIO_2 level of 90%–100%. The other delivery methods listed are not able to provide FIO_2 levels as high. Nasal cannulas deliver a maximum FIO_2 of 44%, simple face masks deliver up to FIO_2 60%, and Venturi masks provide a maximum FIO_2 of 55%. **Focus:** Prioritization

3. **Ans: 1, 2, 6** Checking vital signs and urine output is included in nursing assistant education. An experienced nursing assistant would be able to do this and would know which patient information to report immediately to the supervising RN. A nursing assistant working in the ED setting would also have been trained and know how to establish cardiac monitoring, although dysrhythmia analysis and treatment would be the responsibility of the RN. Obtaining and documenting assessments and starting an IV line should be done by the RN. **Focus:** Delegation

4. **Ans: 1** Although atrial fibrillation at rapid rates can cause a significant drop in cardiac output and blood pressure, the rate of 90–114 is not a likely cause of the patient's hypotension. Ongoing cardiac rhythm monitoring is necessary. Lidocaine would be used if the patient had ventricular dysrhythmias such as premature ventricular contractions or ventricular tachycardia. Adenosine is used to treat paroxysmal supraventricular tachycardia, but is not effective for atrial fibrillation **Focus:** Prioritization

5. **Ans: 2** The ABGs indicate that the patient is hypoxemic (low PaO_2 and oxygen saturation) and has a severe uncompensated respiratory acidosis (low pH and elevated $PaCO_2$). Because she is unable to maintain adequate oxygenation and ventilation independently, mechanical ventilation would be indicated. Administration of sodium bicarbonate is used only if there is a metabolic acidosis. Although she will need ongoing respiratory monitoring and may also benefit from albuterol therapy, these therapies are not adequate in a patient with these severe ABG abnormalities. **Focus:** Prioritization

6. **Ans: 5, 4, 3, 1, 9, 6, 7, 2, 8** The need for intubation should be explained to the patient and family. The patient should be placed supine with the head and neck in the "sniffing" position just prior to intubation, because lying flat usually increases dyspnea. The patient should be pre-oxygenated for 3–5 minutes prior to the intubation attempt. The onset of midazolam effect starts in 1–5 minutes. Inflation of the ET tube cuff is needed for effective ventilation. After bilateral audible breath sounds indicate that the ET tube is above the carina, the tube should be secured prior to obtaining a chest x-ray to confirm optimal placement. **Focus:** Prioritization

7. **Ans: 4** The blood pressure (BP) indicates that systemic tissue perfusion will not be adequate, so measures to improve the BP need to be implemented rapidly. The second priority is to treat the infection that is a likely cause of the temperature elevation and hypotension. The crackles heard in the patient's left lung do not need immediate intervention, because her oxygen saturation is 93%. The decreased pulses are associated with the hypotension and will improve if BP is increased. **Focus:** Prioritization

8. **Ans: 1, 3, 4, 5, 6, 7** The decreased BP and increased heart rate are indicators of shock. The elevation in temperature suggests that sepsis (and massive vasodilation) may be the cause of the shock. The blood-streaked and cloudy urine and back/abdominal pain point to a urinary tract infection (UTI) and/or pyelonephritis as the cause of the sepsis. Diabetics are at increased risk for UTI and sepsis. Slurred speech and atrial fibrillation are not indicators of septic shock. **Focus:** Prioritization

9. **Ans: 2, 3, 1, 4** Ms. D's minimal urine volume with the catheterization and her history of not taking in fluids indicate that she is hypovolemic. In addition, the bacterial toxins released when a patient is septic cause massive vasodilation, which leads to hypotension and decreased tissue perfusion, so increasing the circulating volume is essential for this patient. The dopamine infusion should be started next, to counteract the circulatory vasodilation. The blood cultures (and any other ordered cultures) should be drawn before the antibiotics are started. All of these orders should be implemented rapidly, because septic shock quickly leads to multiple organ dysfunction syndrome (MODS), which is usually fatal. **Focus:** Prioritization

10. **Ans: 3** The most common complication of too-rapid intravenous infusion of fluids is heart failure caused by volume overload. Although peripheral edema, decreased urine output, and jugular venous distention may be indicators that heart failure is developing, they do not occur as rapidly as the back-up of fluids into the pulmonary capillaries and then into the alveoli. **Focus:** Prioritization

11. **Ans: 4** High doses of dopamine are sympathomimetic and increase cardiac conduction and automaticity. The elevated heart rate for this patient will increase her cardiac workload and may cause cardiac ischemia. The BP increase is a therapeutic effect of dopamine. The changes in respiratory rate and oxygen saturation require intervention, but would not be caused by dopamine infusion. **Focus:** Prioritization

12. **Ans: 3** The physiologic effect of dopamine depends on the dose being infused. Low doses (less than 5 mcg/kg/minute) cause renal artery vasodilation, moderate doses (5 to 10 mcg/kg/minute) stimulate myocardial contractility and increase cardiac output, and high doses (greater than 10 mcg/kg/minute) stimulate alpha-receptors, causing vasoconstriction. For this patient, the primary effect of the dopamine is vasoconstriction. Dopamine does bind to receptors in the brain, but this does not affect blood pressure. **Focus:** Prioritization

13. **Ans: 1, 4** LPNs are educated and licensed to perform skills such as monitoring and documentation of intake and output, bedside blood glucose monitoring, and administration of insulin under the supervision of an RN. Although LPNs can collect data about patients, the other assessments and patient care activities listed in the question would require more education and are RN-level skills. **Focus:** Delegation

14. **Ans: 3** The decrease in PA pressures indicates that the patient is still hypovolemic and will need an increase in IV fluids. The arterial BP is improved and you already have an order to increase the dopamine if needed. The atrial fibrillation rate is not dangerously elevated. Although the patient's temperature still is elevated, it has decreased from the previous reading. **Focus:** Prioritization

15. **Ans: 2** The elevated glucose will require that you administer the ordered lispro insulin using the hospital

standard sliding scale insulin orders. The other abnormalities indicate the need for continued monitoring, but will not require any immediate action at this time. **Focus:** Prioritization

16. **Ans: 1** The traveler RN has the required ICU experience to care for this complex case and has been working at the hospital long enough to be familiar with how to obtain supplies, communicate with other departments, and the like. The other nurses either lack experience in caring for critically ill intensive care patients (the new graduate and the PACU nurse), or will not be able to offer the continuity of care that is desirable for the patient. **Focus:** Assignment

Case Study 15: Mitral Valve Disease and Shortness of Breath, pages 159–162

1. **Ans: 3** The client's symptoms indicate acute hypoxemia, so improving oxygen delivery is the priority action. The other actions also may be appropriate, but not as the initial action. **Focus:** Prioritization

2. **Ans: 1** The client's symptoms of hypoxemia and pink frothy sputum and her history of increasing shortness of breath and mitral valve regurgitation point toward pulmonary edema (severe left ventricular failure) as a probable diagnosis. (She also has symptoms of right ventricular failure, but these are not as great a concern.) The client history does not indicate that the client has pulmonary hypertension, so cor pulmonale is not a likely concern. Myocardial infarction may be a precipitating cause for pulmonary edema, but the acute dyspnea is the first concern for treatment. The client's symptoms are not consistent with pulmonary embolus. **Focus:** Prioritization

3. **Ans: 2** The client is hypoxemic, so giving oxygen at the highest level possible is the priority. Calling the physician and administration of morphine are also appropriate actions. Coughing and deep breathing are not likely to be helpful, because they will not clear fluid from the alveoli. **Focus:** Prioritization

4. **Ans: 4** The best clinical indicators of sudden changes in cardiac output are vital signs such as blood pressure, pulse, and respiratory rate. The other data may also be useful in determining how well the client is perfusing, but they are not as important as the blood pressure and pulse rates. **Focus:** Prioritization

5. **Ans: 3** Before the furosemide can be administered, it is essential to know what the client's potassium level is, because the PVCs indicate ventricular irritability, which can be caused by hypokalemia. The digoxin level and retention catheter also are appropriate interventions, but the priority for the client is to ensure that her potassium level is within normal limits and then administer the diuretic to decrease her volume overload. **Focus:** Prioritization

6. **Ans: Insert #16 French Foley catheter** LPN/LVN education and scope of practice include insertion of catheters. Administration of IV medications in unstable clients is best accomplished by RNs who have experience in caring for critically ill clients. Obtaining blood for laboratory tests is usually done by laboratory staff. **Focus:** Delegation

7. **Ans: 4** Morphine is used in pulmonary edema because the venous dilation it causes decreases venous return to the heart and reduces ventricular preload. Although morphine is used to treat angina, this client has not complained of chest pain. Morphine may decrease Ms. C.'s respiratory rate, but this is not a desired effect. Morphine is not a first-line sedative for intubation, and sedation would not be given until just before the client is intubated. **Focus:** Prioritization

8. **Ans: 2** Administration of KCl at a rate no faster than 20 mEq/hour is recommended. Although it is important to increase the client's potassium level quickly, administration of KCl over 1 minute or 10 minutes could lead to cardiac arrest. Administration of the KCl over 8 hours would delay the administration of the furosemide and also leave the client vulnerable to continued dysrhythmias. **Focus:** Prioritization

9. **Ans: 4** Because the client's major problem is pulmonary edema, the most useful information will be changes in her lung sounds. The other information is also helpful in assessing for volume overload, but not as pertinent to the diagnosis of pulmonary edema. **Focus:** Prioritization

10. **Ans: 3** Because nesiritide causes vasodilation and diuresis, hypotension is the most common adverse effect. Systolic blood pressure less than 90 mm Hg is a contraindication for nesiritide infusion. The other data will also be useful in determining whether the client status is improving, but are not as important as frequent blood pressure measurement. **Focus:** Prioritization

11. **Ans: 1** An RN with experience on a coronary stepdown unit would be familiar with the care for clients with left ventricular failure. You have not had an opportunity to evaluate the knowledge level of the agency RN; in addition, this RN will not be familiar with hospital or CCU policies, location of supplies, and so on. The experienced CCU nurse is caring for a client who is potentially very unstable, leaving little time to assess and intervene for Ms. C. The new graduate is not experienced enough to care for a client like Ms. C. whose condition still may deteriorate. The new graduate could be teamed with a more experienced nurse in order to learn more about the care of clients with severe left ventricular failure. **Focus:** Assignment

12. **Ans: 2** Dysrhythmias and visual disturbances are symptoms of digoxin toxicity, a common problem in clients taking digoxin. Digoxin toxicity can lead to fatal dysrhythmias such as ventricular tachycardia and ventricular fibrillation, so a digoxin level should be ordered. The other findings would not be unusual in a client with chronic heart failure and mitral valve disease, although ongoing assessments are indicated. **Focus:** Prioritization

13. **Ans: Furosemide and digoxin** Because you are concerned that the client may have digoxin toxicity, you should hold the digoxin. Hypokalemia can contribute to the risk for digoxin toxicity, and Ms. C. is not acutely short of breath, so the furosemide should also be held until you check with Ms. C.'s doctor. There are no indications that the other medications are causing any adverse effects, so they should all be administered. **Focus:** Prioritization

14. **Ans: 1, 3, 7** Daily weights are an excellent means of monitoring volume status. Clients should be taught to call the doctor (or other provider) when symptoms first begin to worsen, rather than waiting until they need to be admitted to the hospital. ACE inhibitors such as captopril can cause orthostatic hypotension, so changing positions slowly is important in order to avoid dizziness and falls. A weight gain of 2 or 3 pounds

in a day is an indication of volume overload. Ms. C. should be taught to notify the physician if her pulse is less than 60, not just hold the digoxin, because she still may need the inotropic effect of the medication. Furosemide should not be taken in the evening, because it will affect sleep quality. High fluid intake can cause volume overload in clients with heart failure. **Focus:** Prioritization

15. **Ans: 1**   It is important that clients with heart failure be taught that when therapy with beta-blockers is started, symptoms such as weight gain and fatigue may get worse. As the client takes the medication for a longer period, these symptoms should resolve. The client's bradycardia is also an expected effect of carvedilol. If clients are not told to expect these symptoms, they may discontinue the beta-blocking medications. The other actions are not indicated, based on Ms. C.'s assessment. **Focus:** Prioritization

Case Study 16: Multiple Patients with Peripheral Vascular Disease, pages 163–165

1. **Ans: 5, 4, 2, 6, 1, 3**   The worsening back pain of Mr. S. may signal an abdominal aortic aneurysm (AAA) that is enlarging and he is at risk for rupture, which is urgent and immediately life-threatening. Ms. Q's hypertension should be assessed next as she is at risk for complications such as stroke. Next, the patient with the severe pain should be assessed and given pain medication. The patient scheduled for Doppler studies may have questions and need teaching prior to the procedure. The patient with Raynaud's disease should be assessed although the symptoms she is complaining of are typical of this problem. Finally you should see Mr. Z. to discuss arranging for someone to talk with him about smoking cessation. **Focus:** Prioritization

2. **Ans: 2**   You must avoid palpating the abdomen because the mass may be tender and there is a risk of causing a rupture. Auscultating for a bruit and observing for pulsation are appropriate assessment. Pain assessment is appropriate as these patients typically experience steady, gnawing abdominal, flank, or back pain that is unaffected by movement and may last for hours or days. **Focus:** Supervision/prioritization

3. **Ans: 3**   The patient's symptoms and your assessment findings indicate an AAA that may be expanding and this places the patient at risk of rupture. This is an urgent situation and the physician should be notified immediately. You should not place the patient in a high sitting position because this may place added pressure on the patient's AAA. **Focus:** Prioritization

4. **Ans: 1**   The LPN/LVN's educational preparation includes insertion of Foley catheters. In some states, LPN/LVNs can insert IV catheters and administer IV drugs, but this is not true of all states and facilities. To perform these actions, the LPN/LVN would need additional education and training. Check the policies in your state and facility. The nursing assistant could be delegated to take the patient's vital signs, with instructions from the nurse about what to report. **Focus:** Delegation/supervision

5. **Ans: 1, 2, 3**   The nursing student should be able to perform teaching about simple concepts such as coughing and taking deep breaths, simple assessments such as peripheral pulses, and administering oral medications. The nurse remains responsible for these actions. The nurse or someone with special training to perform venipuncture should obtain laboratory draws. The patient may have questions about the surgery, so the discussion about the reasons for surgery should be accomplished by an experienced nurse. The nurse could mentor the student by allowing her to be present during the discussion. **Focus:** Delegation/supervision

6. **Ans: 4**   Postoperatively after AAA repair, bowel sounds are usually absent for 2–3 days and patients have an NG tube in place, set at low suction, until bowel sounds return. The nurse should document the finding only, and teach the student that this is to be expected and why. **Focus:** Delegation/supervision, prioritization

7. **Ans: 1**   Administering the patient's blood pressure medications is aimed at correcting the problem. Getting the patient back into bed and reassessing the patient's BP are appropriate actions, but they do not focus on the goal of lowering the patient's blood pressure. **Focus:** Supervision/delegation, prioritization

8. **Ans: 4**   The nurse should intervene when the patient asked to have the docusate held because narcotic analgesics often cause side effects like constipation. The patient needs to be taught about the importance of this medication in preventing unwanted side effects. If the patient has a good reason for refusing the docusate (e.g., he has been having episodes of diarrhea), then the nurse may hold the drug. The other actions are appropriate. Giving the pain medication before the dressing change will make this a less painful procedure. **Focus:** Delegation/supervision

9. **Ans: 2, 3**   Mr. Z.'s condition is stable and the PACU nurse could begin educating him about smoking cessation. The PACU nurse is skilled at blood pressure monitoring and would have no difficulty meeting Ms. Q.'s needs for care. Ms. A. and Ms. C. need the care of a nurse who is experienced in caring for and teaching patients with peripheral vascular disease. **Focus:** Assignment

10. **Ans: 1, 2, 3, 5**   The underlying pathophysiology of Raynaud's disease is vasospasm of the arterioles and arteries of the upper and lower extremities, usually unilaterally. All of the other teaching points are appropriate to share with a patient with Raynaud's disease. **Focus:** Prioritization

11. **Ans: 3, 4**   The nursing assistant can remind and reinforce nursing care that has already been taught by the RN. Assessing and inspecting the patient require additional education and skills appropriate to the RN's scope of practice. **Focus:** Delegation/supervision

12. **Ans: 2**   Heparin at low doses interacts with antithrombin III to inhibit clotting factors, which results in inhibition of fibrin formation. The drug does nothing to an existing clot. **Focus:** Prioritization

13. **Ans: 1**   The nursing assistant's scope of practice and education include actions related to assisting patients with activities of daily living, such as ambulation. Monitoring, assessing, and providing instructions for the patient require additional education and skills, which are part of the RN's scope of practice. **Focus:** Delegation/supervision

14. **Ans: 1, 2, 4, 5**   Placing the patient supine and elevating his foot places the extremity above heart level, which slows arterial blood flow to the foot. All of the other actions are appropriate for the patient with Buerger's disease. **Focus:** Prioritization

15. **Ans: 4**   Although all of these lipid profile findings are abnormal, the HDL cholesterol ("good cholesterol")

is much too low. A desirable HDL cholesterol level is 40 mg/dL in men and 50 mg/dL in women. The other results are of concern and must be attended to, but they are not as excessively abnormal as the HDL. **Focus:** Prioritization

Case Study 17: Respiratory Difficulty After Surgery, pages 167–172

1. **Ans: 3** The marked decrease in oxygen saturation over the last few hours indicates that Mr. E. is developing respiratory complications that will require immediate nursing action. The other information will also require assessment and possible intervention, but not as urgently as the change in his respiratory status. **Focus:** Prioritization

2. **Ans: 2** Antibiotic trough levels are drawn just before the next scheduled dose. Drawing the blood at 9:00 will give a slightly inaccurate trough level. Obtaining blood at 11:30 would be appropriate for assessment of peak gentamicin level. **Focus:** Prioritization

3. **Ans: 2** Oxygen saturations less than 90% indicate hypoxemia, so the most important action is to improve oxygenation. Sitting in a chair usually improves gas exchange because the lungs can expand more easily. Mr. E.'s anxiety is due to hypoxemia, so morphine is not an appropriate intervention for this client. The assessment should be completed after interventions to improve oxygenation have been implemented. **Focus:** Prioritization

4. **Ans: 1** The ABG results indicate that Mr.E. is hypoxemic and has a metabolic acidosis because of a cellular shift to the anaerobic metabolic pathway. These abnormalities should by corrected by increasing the Pao_2 level. The non-rebreather mask is capable of delivering Fio_2 levels up to 95%. He is hyperventilating in response to hypoxemia, so administration of morphine is not indicated. **Focus:** Prioritization

5. **Ans: 3** The increase in white blood cell (WBC) count is an indicator of infection, a major concern in a client who has had a ruptured appendix. The WBC count may indicate that a change in antibiotic therapy is needed. The abnormalities in the other parameters indicate that ongoing CBC monitoring is necessary, but do not require any acute interventions. **Focus:** Prioritization

6. **Ans: 1** An RN with experience in caring for pediatric clients would be familiar with the care of clients with infection and hyperglycemia, including blood glucose monitoring and administration of insulin. The new graduate does not have enough experience to care independently for a client who is still somewhat unstable. Ms. O. will require assessment and interventions before the on-call RN will be able to arrive. The agency RN will not be familiar with the location of supplies or with hospital policies, such as the standard sliding scale insulin protocol. **Focus:** Assignment

7. **Ans: 4** The client's symptoms of worsening hypoxemia even with increases in supplemental oxygen occurring a few days after the initial injury (such as a ruptured appendix) are most consistent with ARDS. The other complications are possible diagnoses for this client, but not as likely as ARDS. **Focus:** Prioritization

8. **Ans: 2** Improving Mr. E.'s oxygenation is the priority goal. Intubation and mechanical ventilation are required to improve oxygenation in clients with ARDS because of the increased work involved in breathing and because the alveolar infiltrates limit the transfer of oxygen to the pulmonary capillaries. The other interventions should be implemented after intubation is accomplished. **Focus:** Prioritization

9. **Ans: 1** A chest x-ray will confirm that the ET tube is correctly placed 3–5 cm above the carina. The initial assessments done after intubation are listening for bilateral breath sounds and observing for symmetrical chest wall movement with ventilation. Disposable CO_2 monitors are frequently used to ensure that the ET tube is not placed in the esophagus. Monitoring of oxygen saturation is useful in assessing response to treatment, but is not the best indicator of correct ET tube placement, especially in severely hypoxemic clients. **Focus:** Prioritization

10. **Ans: 2** The pH and $Paco_2$ indicate that Mr. E. is retaining CO_2, and increasing the respiratory rate will improve the rate at which the lungs can "blow off" CO_2. The therapeutic goal for clients in respiratory failure is to achieve a Pao_2 of 60 mm Hg or more. Increasing the Fio_2 to a higher level may temporarily improve oxygenation, but it is avoided because exposure to high oxygen levels causes alveolar damage. Raising the tidal volume will increase the chance for complications such as pneumothorax. The CMV mode is usually used for clients who are unconscious or paralyzed because it allows the client no control of respirations and is very uncomfortable. **Focus:** Prioritization

11. **Ans: 1, 6, 7** The PAWP and urine output suggest that Mr. E. is hypovolemic, so increasing his IV fluid intake is essential. Nutritional interventions are important in critically ill clients. Enteral feeding is the preferred method for administration of nutrition because nutrient metabolism is better and fewer complications occur than with total parenteral nutrition. Because Mr. E.'s temperature and WBCs are increasing despite receiving gentamicin and ceftriaxone, adding vancomycin is appropriate. Furosemide administration would lead to further dehydration. The client's hypotension and tachycardia are most likely due to dehydration, so norepinephrine and diltiazem would not be ordered. Total parenteral nutrition is used when the enteral route is not possible. **Focus:** Prioritization

12. **Ans: 3** Having a family member at the bedside will decrease the sense of isolation and anxiety that occurs in the ICU environment, especially in clients who cannot easily communicate because of intubation. The other methods listed may also be used. Restraints are sometimes needed in agitated or confused clients, although the need for restraints must be re-evaluated frequently. Many clients do benefit from the use of antianxiety medications, although use of neuromuscular blockade/paralysis is avoided unless absolutely necessary to improve ABGs. Reminding the client frequently not to pull at the ET tube may also be helpful. **Focus:** Prioritization

13. **Ans: 4** Application of suction causes hypoxemia and trauma to the tracheal mucosa. Suction should only be applied to the catheter while it is being withdrawn to minimize these problems. Hyper-oxygenation is necessary prior to suctioning a client who is at risk for hyoxemia; the nurse should be careful to be sure the Fio_2 is returned to the ordered level after completing suctioning. Use of a closed-suction technique helps decrease the cost of suction catheters and is preferred for clients

using positive end-expiratory pressure (PEEP), but an open-suction technique may also be used. Some clients may require sedation or analgesics prior to suctioning. **Focus:** Prioritization

14. **Ans: 1, 3, 5**   LPN/LVN education includes skills such as oral care, monitoring NG tube feedings, and rectal temperatures. An experienced LPN/LVN would know which client data needed to be reported to the supervising RN immediately. Positioning a client is also included in LPN/LVN education; however, placing a client with an endotracheal tube and multiple hemodynamic monitoring lines in a prone position requires multiple staff members and should be supervised by the RN caring for the client. ET tube suctioning may be delegated to an experienced LPN/LVN in some settings, but in an unstable client, suctioning should be done by the RN. Education and hemodynamic monitoring are RN level responsibilities. **Focus:** Delegation

15. **Ans: 1**   When an alarm sounds, assessment should take place in a systematic fashion, starting with the client. Depending on the findings, the other actions may also be necessary. **Focus:** Prioritization

16. **Ans: 2**   The absence of breath sounds on the right and the high pressures needed to ventilate the client suggest a pneumothorax caused by barotrauma associated with positive pressure ventilation and the use of PEEP. Displacement of the ET tube into one side or extubation also may lead to decreased breath sounds, but the ET tube position would change with these. Aspiration pneumonia is a common complication, but does not present with a sudden onset and absent breath sounds. **Focus:** Prioritization

17. **Ans: 3**   With a pneumothorax, there are usually only a few milliliters of blood in the collection chamber, because there is no blood or fluid trapped in the pleural space. The presence of 100 mL of blood indicates that there may have been trauma to the lung during the chest tube insertion. The other data are expected with chest tube insertion and pneumothorax. The air leak should be monitored, and analgesics should be used to control the pain Mr. E. is experiencing. **Focus:** Prioritization

18. **Ans: 4**   Mr. E. has multiple risk factors for acute renal failure, including his dehydration and use of the potentially nephrotoxic antibiotics gentamicin and vancomycin. Renal failure is one of the common complications of ARDS. The other laboratory data are also abnormal, but do not indicate a need for a change in therapy at present. **Focus:** Prioritization

Notes

Notes

Notes

Notes